Progress in Hepatology Volume 1

Cellular and Molecular Biology

Progress in Hepatology Volume 1

Cellular and Molecular Biology

Proceedings of the 'Takahashi Memorial Forum', held in Tokyo, Japan on 5 November, 1994

Editors:

Masami Yamanaka
Teikyo University School of Medcine
Tokyo, Japan

Kazuhiko Okabe
St. Marianna University School of Medicine
Kanagawa, Japan

Gotaro Toda
The Jikei University School of Medicine
Tokyo, Japan

Associate Editors:

Mikio Zeniya
The Jikei University School of Medicine
Tokyo, Japan

Hajime Takikawa
Teikyo University School of Medicine
Tokyo, Japan

Shoichi Suemori
St. Marianna University School of Medicine
Kanagawa, Japan

1995

Elsevier

Amsterdam – Lausanne – New York – Oxford – Shannon – Tokyo

International Congress Series Volume 1086
ISBN 0-444-82099-x

This book is printed on acid-free paper.

Published by:
Elsevier Science B.V.
P.O. Box 211
1000 AE Amsterdam
The Netherlands

In order to ensure rapid publication this volume was prepared using a method of electronic text processing known as Optical Character Recognition (OCR). Scientific accuracy and consistency of style were handled by the author. Time did not allow for the usual extensive editing process of the Publisher.

Printed in the Netherlands

Preface

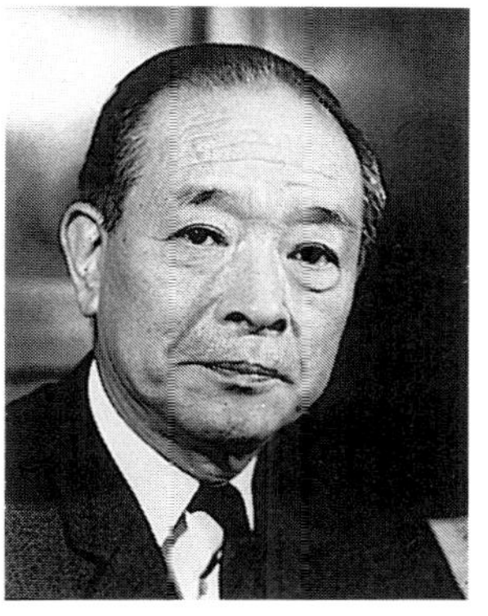

This volume, entitled '*Progress in Hepatology*', is a reflection upon the most recent experiences in Japanese research. Most of the work was presented at a meeting, held in Tokyo, in memory of Tadao Takahashi M.D., Professor Emeritus of the Jikei University School of Medicine, who was one of the founders of the Japanese Association for the Study of the Liver. He chaired the Presidency of the Japanese Association for the Study of the Liver for a long time, and helped develop Japanese hepatology. The reader will find a brief biography in the first chapter of the book. His contribution to the field was outstanding. This meeting, namely the '*Takahashi Memorial Forum*', has been held in the memory of his work, and was intended to represent a milestone in the development of hepatology in Japan.

The editor asked all distinguished hepatologists who had worked with Professor Takahashi to attend a one-day meeting in his memory. Many distinguished hepatologists attended, and unreserved participation was given on all sides. We wish to express our sincere thanks to all contributors to this volume.

This book initially intended to cover recent advances of hepatology in Japan. As the reader may notice, this volume is entitled '*Progress in Hepatology Vol. 1, Cellular and Molecular Biology*'. We plan to publish annually other volumes, focusing on different subject areas in hepatology, particularly in Japan. We hope each volume of this series will be a milestone, as well as an update, in the progression of both clinical and basic studies in hepatology.

We hope this book, and the subsequent series, will create a core annual publication for introducing the work being carried out in Japan to the rest of the world.

Finally, the editors would like to thank all of those at Elsevier Science B.V. who have been vigorously involved in the very rapid publication of this book.

Masami Yamanaka
Professor of Medicine
Teikyo University School of Medicine

In Memoriam
Professor Tadao Takahashi

The late Professor Tadao Takahashi was a great celebrity, unforgettable for Japanese researchers in gastroenterology and hepatology.

He was born on the 31st of August, 1908, at Nihonbashi, a commercial region of Tokyo, the second son of Ren and Chobei Takahashi, who worked as cotton wholesalers. From early childhood he was bright and talented, and he entered the First High School after graduation from the First Junior High School of Tokyo. Directly afterwards he entered the Faculty of Medicine at the Imperial University of Tokyo. To follow such a career was very elitist in those times, and it has been reported that his teacher at the junior high strongly recommended the course to his parents, who had been hoping that he would carry on the family business of wholesaling. His elder brother became a famous economist and a professor at Hitotsubashi University; the brothers played active roles in their respective, although very different, fields of economics and medicine.

After graduating from the Faculty of Medicine at the Imperial University of Tokyo, in March 1932, Professor Tadao Takahashi started to work in the Bacteriology Section of the National Institute for Infectious Diseases (which is now the Institute of Medical Science at the University of Tokyo). After one year, he moved to the First Department of Internal Medicine, in the Faculty of Medicine of the Imperial University of Tokyo, whose Director was Professor Junjiro Shimazono, his father-in-law, and started his career as a researcher in clinical medicine and, making steady progress, he majored in gastroenterology and hepatology. He made a great contribution to the pathogenesis of ascites, hepatic protein metabolism, hematologic disorders in liver cirrhosis, vitamins and the liver, and experimental liver injury including animal models of liver cirrhosis, and he was promoted to the post of Associate Professor despite his comparatively young age. In 1958, he became chairman and professor of the First Department of Medicine, at the Jikei University School of Medicine. Here he developed further his fields of research, aided by his abundant talent and excellent insight. His lectures, particularly the history of research on the pathogenesis of disease and pathophysiology, deeply impressed students, and many of them entered the First Department of Medicine.

During his career as a professor of medicine, he became the president of many Japanese medical societies, such as the Japanese Society of Gastroenterology and the Japanese Society of Hepatology. Furthermore, he served as the general secretary of the Third World Congress of Gastroenterology held in Tokyo in 1966, and he contributed greatly to the management of the Third Meeting of the International Association for the Study of the Liver that was held at the same time under the presidency of Dr Hans Popper.

In addition, he worked as chairman of the board of directors of the Japanese Society of Gastroenterology from April 1966 to March 1988, and as the first chairman of the board of directors of the Japanese Society of Hepatology, founded in July 1965. As the chairman of the board of directors (until July 1980) he made great efforts in founding the management of the Japanese Society of Hepatology, in which doctors in both basic and clinical medicine coordinate the progress being made in research.

Dr Tadao Takahashi was a very shrewd, foresighted and instructive man. Furthermore, he was also a very refined 'dandy' of a man, often seen of people born in a big city such as Tokyo. These characteristics made him an engaging leader. Many professors of gastroenterology and hepatology have been guided by Professor Takahashi, a most distinguished clinician and medical researcher.

Professor Tadao Takahashi had various hobbies, such as skiing, mountain photography, music, and theatre. His mountain photographs of Europe, which he often visited after the Second World War, are alive in the memories of many people, together with his humorous and enjoyable speeches.

Due to his career and personality, Dr Tadao Takahashi had many friends in various fields, not just in the medical world, but also in politics, finance and the world of entertainment. He was known as the physician in charge of the famous actors of Kabuki, which is one of the classical forms of Japanese entertainment.

Professor Tadao Takahashi died of penumonia on the 23rd of November, 1987. Although, at 79 years of age, he was in the late autumn of his life, many people were greatly saddened by his death.

Contents

Progress in Hepatology Vol. 1.
Cellular and Molecular Biology.
M. Yamanaka, K. Okabe and G. Toda, editors.

Molecular structure and pathophysiological roles of intercellular junctions in the liver

Michio Mori,[1] Yun Zhong,[1] Katsuhiko Enomoto,[2] Masahito Oyamada,[1] and Norimasa Sawada[1]

[1]The 2nd Department of Pathology, Sapporo Medical University School of Medicine, Sapporo, Japan; [2]Present address: The 1st Department of Pathology, Akita University School of Medicine, Akita, Japan

Abstract. Hepatocytes tightly connect with each other by cell junctions to form liver cell plates, which compose the parenchyma of the liver. Among the intercellular junctions, tight junctions function as an occluding apparatus which serves as a barrier to the movement of water and ions, thus preventing bile from leaking from the canaliculi into the blood. A novel tight junction-associated protein, 7H6 antigen, was identified in our laboratory and shown to have crucial roles in the maintenance of barrier function of tight junctions. On the other hand, gap junctions link directly neighboring hepatocytes and thus function as a communicating apparatus. Roles of gap junctions in the ordered contraction of the bile canaliculi were indicated. Significance of these junctions in the physiological liver function and changes in the junctions under pathological conditions of the liver such as acute focal necrosis, regenerative proliferation and hepatocarcinogenesis was discussed.

Key words: cell-cell communication, gap junction, hepatocarcinogenesis, permeability barrier, regenerating liver, tight junction.

Introduction

Most cells in the human body are organized into co-operative assemblies by connecting with each other with intercellular junctions. Epithelial cells are tightly bound together into sheets with specialized cell junctions, and line all the cavities of the body, whereas endothelial cells bound into sheets with cell junctions line the cavities of blood and lymphatic vessels. These sheets serve as a barrier to the movement of water, solutes, and cells from one body compartment to another. On the other hand, epithelial cells constituting organs communicate with each other via cell junctions to perform the organized function of the organ.

Cell junctions can be classified into the following three groups according to

Address for correspondence: Michio Mori, M.D., Professor of Pathology, Sapporo Medical University, School of Medicine, S.1, W.17, Chuo-ku, Sapporo 060, Japan. Fax: 81-11-011-613-5665.

their functions: 1) occluding junctions (tight junctions), which prevent small molecules from leaking from one side of the cells to the other; 2) anchoring junctions (adherent junctions, desmosomes), which mechanically attach cells to their neighbors; and 3) communicating junctions (gap junctions, chemical synapses), which mediate the passage of chemicals and signals from one cell to the neighbors.

In this brief review, we will summarize the recent data on tight junctions and gap junctions mainly obtained in our laboratory, in an attempt to elucidate the roles of cell junctions in the physiology and pathology of the liver.

Molecular structure and physiological function of the tight junction

Tight junctions are most important for the selective permeability barrier function of epithelial and endothelial cells, but the constituents of the junction and the mechanisms by which the barrier function is regulated have not been fully clarified [1]. To understand the molecular structure of tight junctions, it is first necessary to define the molecular components of the junction. Recent studies have identified several proteins associated with the cytoplasmic side of tight junctions by monoclonal antibodies against cell junction-rich membrane fractions. These include ZO-1 [2], ZO-2 [3], cingulin [4], 7H6 antigen [5], 130 kD protein [6], rab13 [7], and 220 kD protein [8].

More recently, an integral membrane protein, "occludin", preferentially localized at tight junctions was identified [9]. Nevertheless, none of the molecules has so far been shown to be responsible for the barrier function of tight junctions.

The 7H6 antigen is a tight junction-associated protein recently identified in our laboratory with a monoclonal antibody (7H6) generated against a bile canaliculus-rich membrane fraction prepared from rat liver [5]. The antigen was shown to localize by immunofluorescent microscopy at the junctional complex regions of hepatocytes (Fig. 1) and other epithelia, and was shown by immunogold electron microscopy to localize at the cytoplasmic side of tight junctions (Fig. 2). Immunoblot analysis of a bile canaliculus-rich fraction of rat liver using 7H6, anti-ZO-1 antibody (R26,4C), and anti-cingulin antibody revealed that 7H6 reacts selectively with a 155 kD protein, whereas anti-ZO-1 antibody reacts only with a 225 kD protein. Anti-cingulin antibody reacted solely with 140 and 108 kD proteins. Immunoprecipitation of detergent extracts obtained from metabolically labeled Madin-Darby canine kidney (MDCK) cells with anti-ZO-1 antibody co-precipitated a 160 kD, ZO-2 protein with ZO-1 as reported by Gumbiner et al. [3], but not with the 7H6 antigen. Therefore, we concluded that 7H6 antigen is a novel tight junction-associated protein immunologically distinct from ZO-1, ZO-2 and cingulin.

The 7H6 antigen was also shown to be different from other tight

Fig. 1. Immunofluorescent localization of 7H6 antigen in a frozen section of rat liver. The antigen localizes preferentially at the junctional complex regions along the bile canaliculi. Bar, 20 μm.

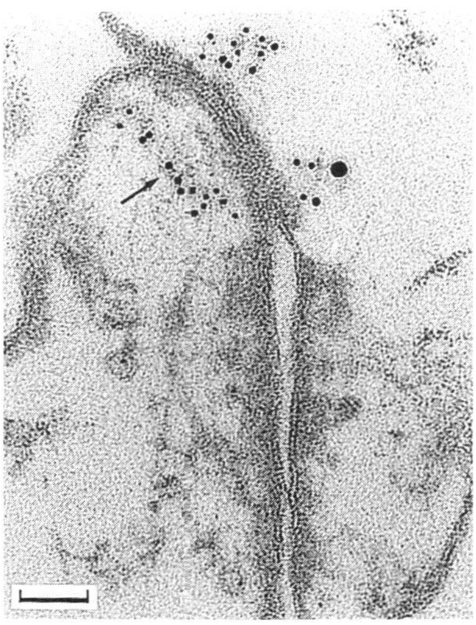

Fig. 2. Immunoelectron microscopic localization of 7H6 antigen in the bile canaliculus-rich fraction of rat liver. Immunogold particles localize preferentially along the cytoplasmic side of the tight junction. Bar, 20 μm.

junction-associated proteins in that the antigen is expressed only at tight junctions of epithelial cells, whereas other tight junction proteins were reported to be expressed at tight junctions of both epithelial and endothelial cells. Further extensive immunofluorescent studies showed that 7H6 antigen is expressed in the endothelial cells of microvessels in the brain. It is well known that the vascular endothelial cells have rather more leaky tight junctions than epithelial cells except for those in the brain microvessels, in which tight junctions are resistant to the passage of ions and macromolecules which account for the most prominent structural constituent of the blood-brain barrier (BBB) [10]. Therefore, we speculated that the expression of 7H6 antigen at tight junctions might reflect the integrity of tight junctions that modulate the barrier function. The barrier function of tight junctions can be assessed by measuring electrical transepithelial resistance (TER) using microelectrodes, which shows the resistance to current flowing and hence its ionic permeability. The barrier function can also be assayed by measuring the amount of small extracellular tracer molecules at the lower chamber which were added above the cell monolayers grown on the filter culture insert of Ussing's double chamber.

7H6 antigen expression and barrier function of endothelial cells

To assess whether the expression of 7H6 antigen at tight junctions has any correlation with the permeability barrier function of endothelial cells, we examined the effects of retinoic acid (RA) or cAMP on the expression of 7H6 antigen and the barrier function of rat lung endothelial (RLE) cells in vitro. RLE cells in a confluent density expressed ZO-1 at tight junctions, but did not express 7H6 antigen at least as far as immunofluorescent microscopy is concerned (Fig. 3). Under such a condition, RLE cells were highly permeable to albumin (permeability coefficient $= 4.6 \times 10^{-6}$ cm/s) (Fig. 4) with low TER (22 ohm/cm^2). When these cells were cultured for a few days with 10^{-5} M all-trans RA or 0.5 mM dibutyryl cAMP, the cells expressed 7H6 antigen at tight junctions as ZO-1 (Fig. 3). The expression of 7H6 antigen was associated with an increase in TER (up to 50.33 ohm/cm^2) with concomitant decrease in permeability to albumin (permeability coefficient $= 2.2 \times 10^{-6}$ cm/s) (Fig. 4), indicating that 7H6 antigen expression at tight junctions correlates with the development of endothelial barrier function.

7H6 antigen expression and barrier function of epithelial cells

We then examined the relationship between the epithelial barrier function and the expression of 7H6 antigen at tight junctions. For this purpose, we utilized MDCK cells in a confluent density which expressed both 7H6 antigen

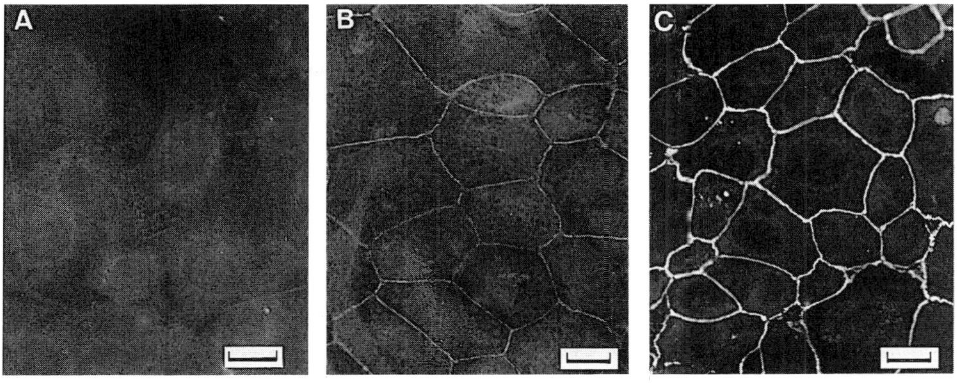

Fig. 3. Immunofluorescent localization of 7H6 antigen (A and B) and ZO-1 (C) in RLE cells in a confluent density. Data shown for control RLE monolayers (A and C), as well as monolayers treated with retinoic acid for 4 days (B). Bar, 10 μm.

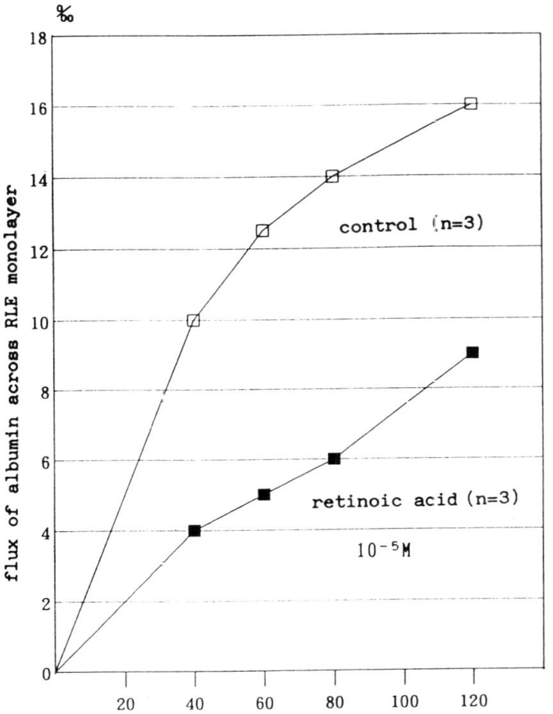

Fig. 4. Effects of retinoic acid on the permeability of RLE cells to albumin. Results are expressed as the mean ±SEM.

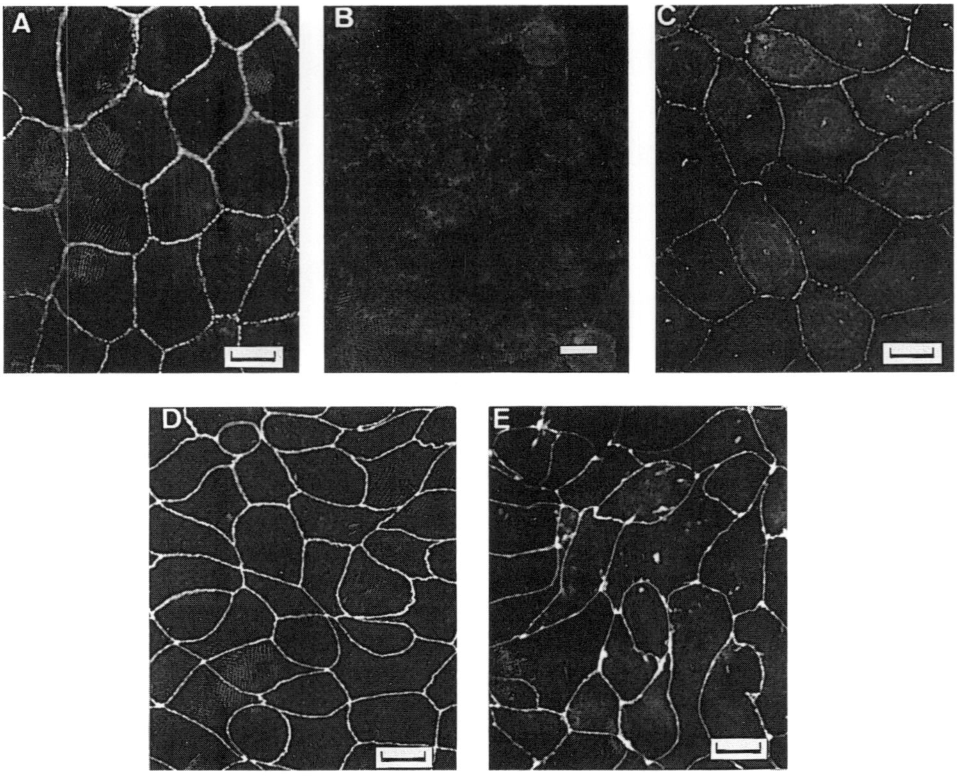

Fig. 5. Immunofluorescent localization of 7H6 antigen (A, B and C) and ZO-1 (D and E) in MDCK cells in a confluent density. Data shown for control MDCK monolayers (A and D), as well as monolayers treated with the metabolic inhibitors for 30 min (B and E), and 3 hrs after removal of the inhibitors (C). Bar, 10 μm.

and ZO-1 at tight junctions [11] (Fig. 5). The cells maintained a tight barrier function as determined by resistance to electron-dense lanthanum permeation at electron microscopic level and extremely high TER (1,500 ohm/cm^2). When the MDCK cells were treated with a combination of metabolic inhibitors (10 mM antimycin A and 10 mM 2-deoxyglucose), tight junctions became permeable to the tracer with a dramatic decrease in TER (below 100 ohm/cm^2) within 30 min (Fig. 6). Treatment of the cells with metabolic inhibitors altered neither cell viability nor the ultrastructure of the cells, yet the 7H6 antigen disappeared from tight junctions as the junctions became permeable to lanthanum (Fig. 5). On the other hand, no significant changes in the immunofluorescent localization of ZO-1 were observed, consistent with the observation that the localization and content of ZO-1 are identical in two strains of MDCK cells which differ significantly in tight junction permeability

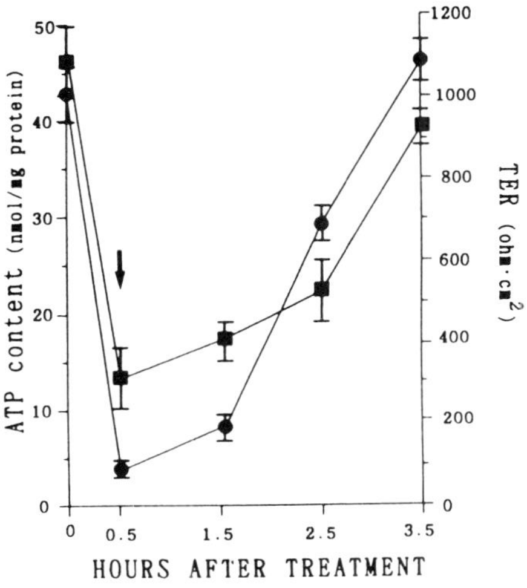

Fig. 6. Effects of the metabolic inhibitors on the ATP (■) content and TER (●) of MDCK cells. The arrow indicates the point when the metabolic inhibitors are removed. Results are expressed as the mean ±SEM.

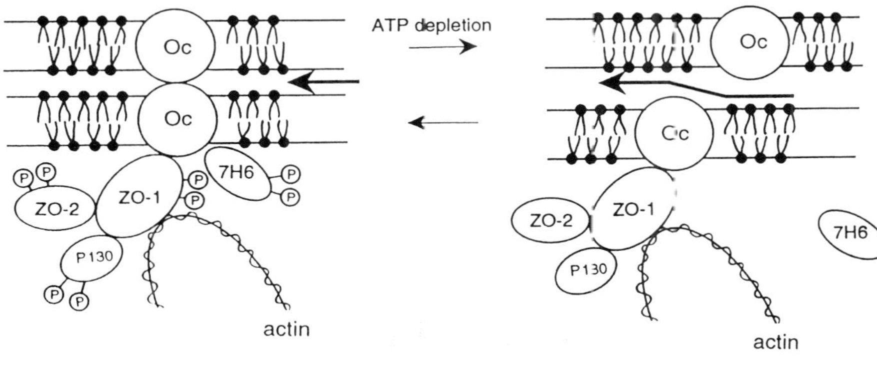

Fig. 7. A hypothetical molecular model for the permeability barrier of tight junctions.

[12]. The 7H6 antigen appeared at tight junctions again as TER recovered to a high level (1,500 ohm/cm^2) within 3 h after withdrawal of metabolic inhibitors. The disappearance of 7H6 antigen from tight junctions under ATP-depleted conditions is unlikely to be due to epitope alteration or degradation of 7H6 molecules, because immunoblot analysis showed that the amount of 7H6 antigen in the whole homogenates of the MDCK cells was virtually unaltered by ATP depletion. Therefore, we consider that 7H6 molecules aggregate at tight junctions under ATP-supplemented conditions and disperse from the junctions under ATP-depleted conditions. The 7H6

antigen is shown to be phosphorylated at the tyrosine residue under ATP-supplemented conditions like other tight junction-associated proteins. On the other hand, 7H6 antigen was found not to be phosphorylated when the cellular ATP is depleted, suggesting that phosphorylation of 7H6 antigen is closely related to the localization of this protein at tight junctions.

Molecular mechanisms of barrier function regulation

Such a close correlation between the localization of 7H6 antigen at tight junctions and the maintenance of paracellular permeability in both endothelial and epithelial cells strongly suggested that 7H6 antigen crucially regulates the barrier function of tight junctions. Although the molecular structure of tight junctions has not yet been fully understood, freeze-fracture electron microscopy reveals that an anastomosing network of strands of transmembrane junctional proteins corresponds to tight junctions [13]. Recently Furuse et al. [9] in Tsukita's laboratory found a novel integral membrane protein, occludin, which localized preferentially at tight junctions of endothelial and epithelial cells in chickens. Whether occludin functions as a molecular sieve for ions and small molecules which pass through the paracellular pathway remains to be elucidated, but it is highly plausible that occludin molecules correspond to the transmembrane junctional particles revealed by freeze-fracture electron microscopy. Since our immunogold electron microscopy showed that 7H6 antigen is a cytoplasmic component of tight junctions [5], we hypothesize that 7H6 antigen might bind occludin molecules at tight junctions and thus modulate their conformation to restrict the passage of ions and small molecules (Fig. 7). It is evident that the conclusion must await molecular characterization of the 7H6 antigen. Further studies including cDNA cloning are now in progress in our laboratory.

Changes in the expression of 7H6 antigen in liver diseases

Our preliminary immunohistochemical studies showed that the expression of 7H6 antigen at hepatocyte tight junctions is less prominent in the liver of LEC rats with spontaneous hepatitis [14], suggesting that decrease in the paracellular barrier function is responsible, at least in part, for the development of jaundice. However, this hypothesis has not been proven in vitro, since it is difficult to make hepatocytes to form confluent monolayer sheets on a polycarbonate filter culture insert of Ussing's double chamber. On the other hand, in the liver of rats after acute focal (contrilobular) necrosis due to single intraperitoneal injection of thioacetamide, 7H6 antigen disappeared from hepatocytes undergoing necrosis labeled with intravenously injected propidium iodide. On the contrary, the expression of 7H6 antigen in hepatocytes

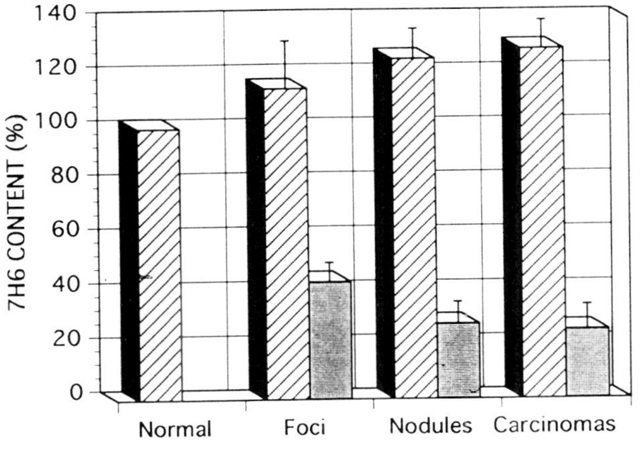

Fig. 8. Changes in the expression of 7H6 antigen during the course of hepatocarcinogenesis in rats. Hatched bars show the expression of 7H6 antigen in the surrounding areas, whereas stippled ones represent that of 7H6 antigen in the preneoplastic and neoplastic liver lesions. Results are expressed as the mean ±SEM.

located in the areas surrounding the necrotic lesions was increased [15]. Such changes in the expression of tight junctions are quite different from those in the expression of gap junctions, which disappear not only from necrotic hepatocytes but also from hepatocytes undergoing restorative proliferation. The significance of such a striking difference in the expression of tight junction protein and gap junction protein remains obscure, but it is likely that enhanced expression of 7H6 antigen fortifies the barrier function of hepatocyte tight junctions to prevent bile from rushing into the circulation. On the other hand, gap junctions disappear not only from injured hepatocytes but also from proliferating hepatocytes as observed in the regenerating liver following partial hepatectomy.

Recently Willott et al. [16] have noted striking sequence homology between the amino-terminal 793 residues of ZO-1, the first tight junction protein cloned and fully sequenced, and a family of proteins implicated in signal transduction at specialized cell junctions. The defining family member is the discs-large (dlg) tumor suppressor of *Drosophila*, located at septate junctions of epithelial cells in the imaginal discs [17]. Since the mutation in the *dlg* gene results in loss of cell polarity and intercellular adhesion, and induces neoplastic proliferation of epithelial cells [17], it is speculated that tight junction proteins act as a tumor suppressor. Immunohistochemical and semiquantitative study in our laboratory has shown that the expression of 7H6 antigen decreases sequentially during the process of hepatocarcinogenesis in rats [18] (Fig. 8).

Roles of gap junctions in liver function

A gap junction is a cluster of transmembrane channels composed of a family of structural proteins named connexins. Gap junctions directly link neighboring cells and mediate exchange of low molecular weight metabolites and ions, including second messengers, cAMP, inositol triphosphate (IP^3) and Ca^{2+} between the cells [19]. At present, more than ten connexins, such as cx43, cx37, cx32, and cx26, have been cloned and divided into two groups based on the sequence homology between two of the four transmembrane domains [20]. In hepatocytes, cx32 and cx26 are expressed. The ratio of cx32 to cx26 is estimated to be 10:1 in isolated liver gap junction plaques [21]. The biological significance of such different expression of cx32 and cx26 is not known. Polyclonal antibodies against cx32 and cx26 generated by immunizing rabbits with synthetic peptides corresponding to the cytoplasmic domain of connexin demonstrated that cx32 is expressed by virtually all hepatocytes throughout the liver lobule, whereas cx26 is expressed by hepatocytes located in the periportal zones. Specificity of the antibody was proven by the fact that the antibody injection into one of the paired hepatocytes in vitro inhibited the transfer of low molecular weight fluorescent dye (Lucifer Yellow) microinjected into the opposite hepatocyte [22].

The liver functions both as an exocrine gland, secreting bile through the bile ducts, and simultaneously as an endocrine gland, releasing a variety of plasma proteins directly into the bloodstream. Thus the structural organization and functional polarity of hepatocytes should be kept highly ordered and integrated. The primary secretion of bile is elaborated into small bile canalicular spaces that are formed as shallow grooves of the plasma membrane between adjacent hepatocytes. Recent studies have revealed that bile canalicular contractions based on pericanalicular actin microfilaments act as a pump to facilitate bile flow in the canalicular system [23]. Endothelin-1 increases the frequency of bile canalicular contraction significantly in a dose-dependent manner under physiological concentrations [24]. A transient increase in the intracellular Ca^{2+} was demonstrated upon the addition of endothelin-1 to the medium, suggesting that the initial increase in cytoplasmic Ca^{2+} ion concentration would trigger the bile canalicular contraction [25]. Confocal laser microscopy of living hepatocyte couplets loaded with Fluo-3 revealed that a transient increase in Ca^{2+} concentration occurs at the rim of contracting bile canaliculus [22].

Recent advances in the fluorescence microscopic techniques have enabled us to show the motility of bile canaliculi in the living rat liver. By combining the use of sodium fluorescein into bile, with digitally enhanced fluorescence microscopy and time-lapse videography, Watanabe et al. [26] have demonstrated that the bile canalicular contraction moves unidirectionally from centrolobular hepatocytes towards the portal bile ducts. Such an ordered pattern of bile canalicular contraction suggests highly integrated mechanisms which entail a high degree of communication between neighboring hepatocytes.

In order to analyze whether the gap junctional communication plays any roles in the ordered contraction of cells, we examined the relationship between the expression of gap junctions and synchronized contraction of cultured rat cardiac myocytes [27]. This is because of the difficulty in the establishment of co-ordinated bile canalicular contraction system of hepatocytes in vitro.

By combining the use of Fura-2 with fluorescence microscopy and a high-sensitive video camera, synchronized elevation in the intracellular concentration of Ca^{2+} in a cluster of cardiac myocytes was demonstrated. Such an elevation of Ca^{2+} was coincident with the synchronized beating which occurs in a cluster of myocytes demonstrated with a Fotonic Sensor. Immunofluorescence microscopy showed that the expression of cx43 (cardiac myocyte connexin) increased with the lapse of culture time, concident with the increase in cell-cell communication measured by dye transfer assay and synchronized beating. Synchronized beating was abolished when heptanol or octanol (which perturb gap junctional cell-cell communication) was added to the culture medium [28]. These results suggested that the cell-cell communication through hepatocyte gap junctions may be responsible for the establishment of ordered contraction of bile canaliculi in the liver.

Changes in expression of gap junction proteins in liver diseases

It has been shown that the expression of gap junction proteins decreases in regenerating liver following partial hepatectomy. Reduction in the expression of connexins occurs soon after partial hepatectomy and reached the lowest level at the time when the hepatocyte proliferation reached the highest level. Cx32 decreased almost in parallel with cx26 (Fig. 9). To the contrary, during the course of hepatocarcinogenesis in rats, the expression of cx32 decreases sequentially in parallel with the progress of carcinogenesis, while leaving the expression of cx26 relatively high (Fig. 10) by the time hepatocellular carcinomas develop [29]. Gap junctional cell-cell communication is shown to be regulated not only at classical regulatory levels, such as transcription, translation and posttranslational modification, but also at cellular levels, such as cell-cell recognition processes [30]. Alterations of such regulatory mechanisms would account for the development of unregulated cell proliferation and altered phenotypes of cancer cells.

Conclusion

The liver acts as the central organ in the metabolism, thus the structural organization of the parenchymal cells into liver cell plates loosely covered

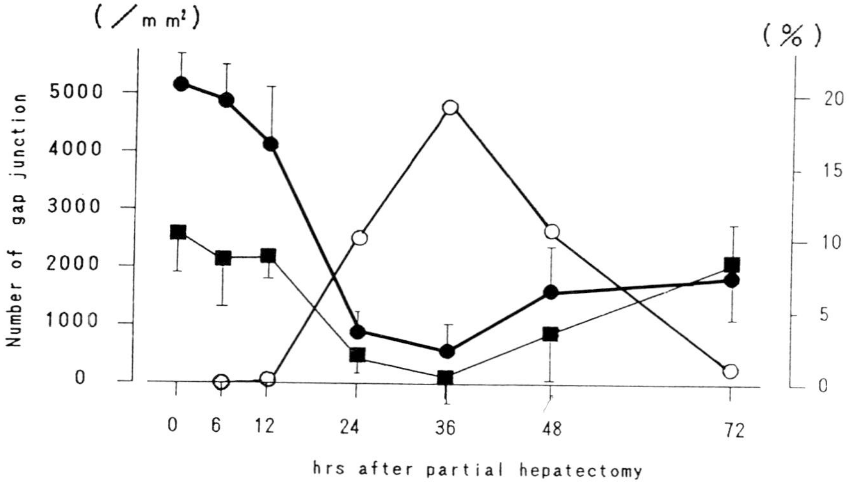

Fig. 9. Changes in the expression of cx32 (●) and cx26 (■) during the course of regeneration following 2/3 partial hepatectomy in rats. Results are expressed as the mean ±SEM.

with fenestrated endothelial sheets are essential for effective uptake of substrates from the circulation and subsequent secretion of plasma proteins into the blood stream. On the other hand, hepatocytes secrete bile constituents into the bile canaliculi and the liver cell plates drained with sinusoidal blood flow yet drain bile towards the bile ducts without leaking it into the circulation. In this paper, we demonstrated the crucial roles of occluding and communicating junctions in the maintenance and regulation of specific liver functions. Further progress in the molecular cell biological studies on cell junctions and cell-cell interactions is expected for the better understanding of the pathobiology of the liver.

Acknowledgement

This study was supported in part by a Grant-in-Aid for Scientific Research from the Ministry of Education, Science and Culture, Japan.

References

1. Anderson JM, Balda MS, Fanning AS. Curr Opin Cell Biol 1993;5:772–778.
2. Stevenson BR et al. J Cell Biol 1986;103:755–766.
3. Gumbiner B, Lowenkopf T, Apatira D. Proc Natl Acad Sci USA 1991;88:3460–3464.
4. Citi S et al. Nature 1988;333:272–275.

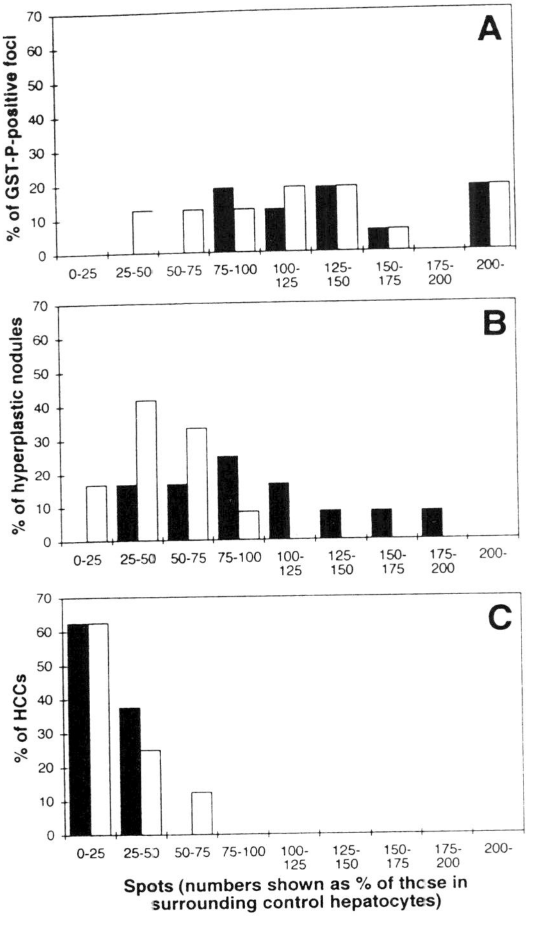

Fig. 10. Changes in the expression of cx32 (open bars) and cx26 (solid bars) in the GST-P-positive foci (A), hyperplastic modules (B) and HCCs (C). Numbers are shown as a percentage of those seen in the surrounding rat liver.

5. Zhong Y et al. J Cell Biol 1993;120:477–483.
6. Jesaitis LA, Goodenough DA. J Cell Biol 1994;124:949–961.
7. Zhraoui A et al. J Cell Biol 1994;124:101–115.
8. Itoh M et al. J Cell Biol 1993;121:491–502.
9. Furuse M et al. J Cell Biol 1993;123:1777–1788.
10. Krause D, Mischeck U, Galla HJ et al. Neurosci Lett 1991;128:301–304.
11. Zhong Y et al. Exp Cell Res 1994;214:614–620.
12. Stevenson BR et al. J Cell Biol 1988;107:2401–2408.
13. Schneeberger EE, Lynch RD. Am J Physiol 1992;262:L647–L661.
14. Mori M et al. Am J Pathol 1994;144:200–204.
15. Kojima T et al. Sequential changes in intercellular junctions between hepatocytes during the course of acute liver injury: restoration after thioacetamide treatment. Virchows Arch (in press).

16. Willott E et al. Proc Natl Acad Sci USA 1993;90:7834–7838.
17. Woods DF, Bryant PJ. Cell 1991;66:451–464.
18. Zhong Y et al. Jpn J Cancer Res 1994;85:351–356.
19. Saez JC et al. Proc Natl Acad Sci USA 1989;86:2708–2712.
20. Willecke K et al. Euro J Cell Biol 1991;56:1–7.
21. Nicholson B et al. Nature 1987;329:732–734.
22. Mori M. J Electron Microsc Electron microscopic and new microscopic studies of hepatocyte cytoskeleton: physiological and pathological relevance. (in press).
23. Phillips MJ et al. Hepatology 1982;2:763–768.
24. Kamimura Y et al. Biochem Biophys Res Comm 1993;191:817–822.
25. Watanabe S, Phillips MJ. Proc Natl Acad Sci USA 1984;81:6164–6168.
26. Watanabe N et al. J Cell Biol 1991;113:1069–1080.
27. Kimura H et al. Comp Biochem Physiol 1993;105C:479–485.
28. Oyamada M et al. Exp Cell Res 1994;212:351–358.
29. Sakamoto H, Oyamada M, Enomoto K et al. Jpn J Cancer Res 1992;83:1210–1215.
30. Jongen WMF, Fitzgerald DJ, Asamoto M et al. J Cell Biol 1991;114:545–555.

Progress in Hepatology Vol. 1.
Cellular and Molecular Biology.
M. Yamanaka, K Okabe and G. Toda, editors.

Transport in the liver and its abnormalities

Hajime Takikawa and Masami Yamanaka
Department of Medicine, Teikyo University School of Medicine, Tokyo, Japan

Abstract. Recent studies have elucidated the mechanisms of the hepatic transport of various compounds. In this chapter, recent advances in this field, especially regarding the hepatic transport of bile acids and organic anions and its abnormalities, are discussed. Bile acids and organic anions are mainly taken up by Na^+-dependent and Na^+-independent transport systems, respectively. Basolateral carriers for bile acids and organic anions have recently been cloned. However, no significant homology was observed between these proteins and previously reported various basolateral liver plasma membrane carriers for bile acids and organic anions. Intrahepatic transport of bile acids and organic anions may be mediated by cytosolic binders and the role of vesicular transport in intrahepatic transport of these compounds remains to be elucidated. Bile acids and organic anions are excreted into the bile by distinct ATP-dependent carriers at the canalicular plasma membrane. Mutant Eisai hyperbilirubinemic rats (EHBRs) with impaired biliary excretion of organic anions may have an abnormal ATP-dependent canalicular organic anion carrier, that has not yet been identified. Various experimental models for intrahepatic cholestasis have been reported and various mechanisms of intrahepatic cholestasis have been postulated. As examples, recent advances in cholestatic rat models induced by ethinylestradiol and lithocholate-3-O-glucuronide are discussed.

Key words: bile acids, cholestasis, cytosolic binders, Eisai hyperbilirubinemic rat (EHBR), ethinylestradiol, lithocholate-3-O-glucuronide, organic anions.

Introduction

Recent studies have contributed to the elucidation of the mechanisms of the hepatic transport of various compounds. In this chapter, recent advances in this field, especially regarding the transport of bile acids and organic anions and its abnormalities, hyperbilirubinemia and cholestasis, will be reviewed.

Three factors have largely contributed to the advances in this field; 1) techniques for the separation of the basolateral and the canalicular plasma membrane vesicles, which are especially useful to study the transport mechanisms at the canalicular membrane, 2) the discovery of hyperbilirubinemic mutant rats, which contributed to the understanding of canalicular organic anion transport, and 3) the introduction of molecular biology

Address for correspondence: Hajime Takikawa, MD, Department of Medicine, Teikyo University School of Medicine, Kaga 2-11-1, Itabashi-ku, Tokyo 173, Japan. Fax: 81-3-3964-5710.

Table 1. Major constituents of hepatic bile (mM)

Electrolytes	
Na^+	140–165
Cl^-	77–117
HCO_3^-	12–55
Ca^{2+}	2.5–6.4
Organic anions	
Bile acids	3–45
Bilirubin	1–2
Lipids	
Phospholipids	140–180 (mg/dl)
Cholesterol	100–320 (mg/dl)
Proteins	2–20 (mg/dl)
Glutathione	3–5

techniques in this field, which on the other hand have raised various controversies against previous works.

Little is known about the mechanisms of intrahepatic cholestasis. Although various mechanisms of cholestasis have been considered, their physiologic importance as causes of cholestasis is not clear. In this chapter, we will discuss the recent advances in cholestatic rat models induced by ethinylestradiol and lithocholate-3-O-glucuronide.

Bile formation

Table 1 summarizes the major constituents of hepatic bile, and Figs. 1 and 2 demonstrate the classification of bile flow and the mechanisms of the hepatic transport of important bile constituents, respectively [1–4]. Among them, bile acids are most important to produce bile acid-dependent canalicular bile flow; the osmotic pressure of bile acids and Na^+, their counter ion, is considered to move water from the sinusoidal space to the canalicular lumen through the tight junction (Fig. 2). Furthermore, bile acids are also important to solubilize cholesterol in the bile as well as phospholipids. Glutathione is considered to be a driving force of bile acid-independent canalicular bile flow because of its high choleretic activity [5,6]. HCO_3^- is important for ductular bile flow which is stimulated by secretin.

Hepatic transport of bile acids and organic anions

Hepatic uptake

Hepatic uptake of bile acid amides is mainly mediated by an Na^+-dependent transport system, which has been examined in the perfused rat liver [7],

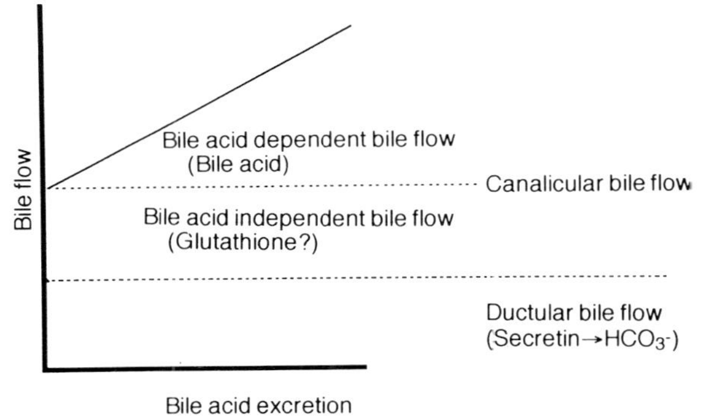

Fig. 1. Relationship between biliary bile acid excretion and bile flow.

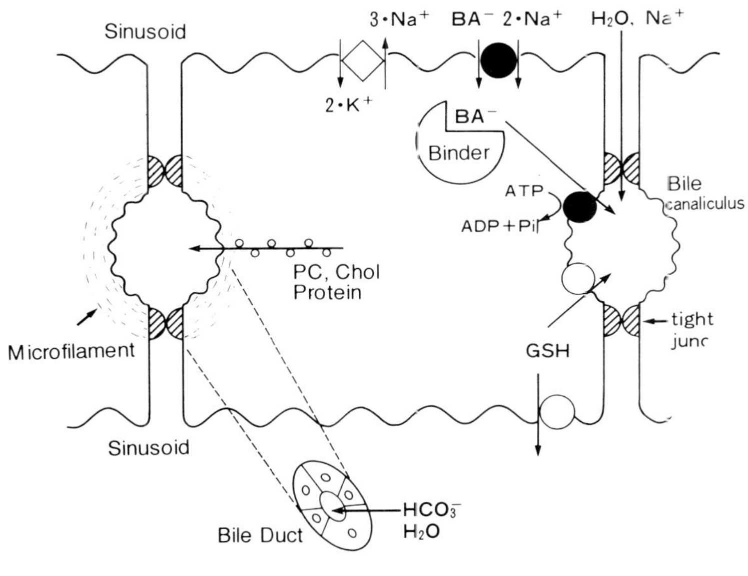

Fig. 2. Mechanisms of hepatic transport. BA, bile acid; PC, phosphatidylcholine; Chol, cholesterol; GSH, reduced glutathione.

isolated or cultured rat hepatocytes [8–10] and rat basolateral liver plasma membrane vesicles [11]. Zimmerli et al. reported the multiplicity of Na^+-dependent taurocholate uptake by basolateral liver plasma membrane vesicles according to inhibition studies using various substrates [12]. Other mechanisms of bile acid uptake include Na^+-independent transport for unconjugated bile acids such as cholate [13], and by a simple diffusion for hydrophobic bile

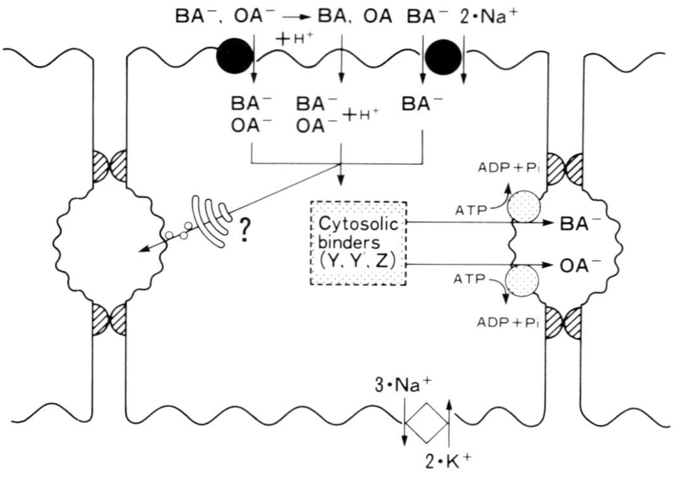

Fig. 3. Hepatic transport of bile acids and organic anions. BA, bile acid; OA, organic anions.

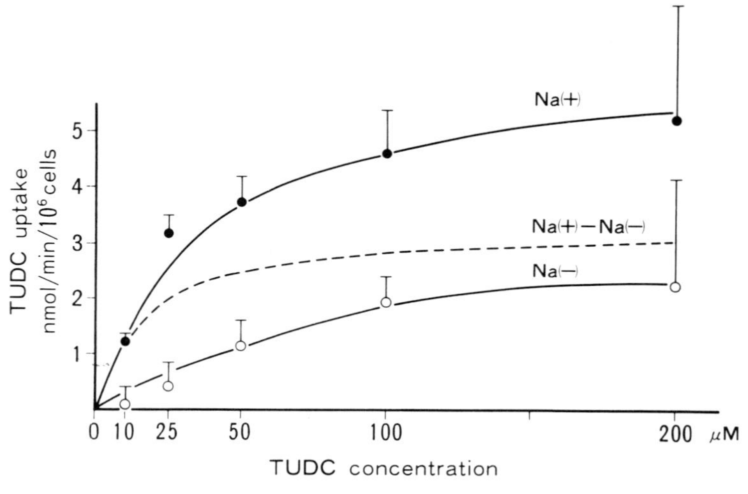

Fig. 4. Initial uptake of tauroursodeoxycholate (TUDC) by freshly isolated rat hepatocytes in the presence and absence of Na^+ ion in the medium [10]. The dotted line represents a simulation of Na^+-dependent TUDC uptake.

acids such as lithocholate [9,14]. Figure 4 shows the tauroursodeoxycholate uptake by isolated rat hepatocytes. The Na^+-dependent uptake is important at low substrate concentrations and the Na^+-independent uptake may have a role at higher substrate concentrations.

Von Dippe and Levy [15] reported the purification of a 48 kDa Na^+-dependent bile acid carrier from the rat basolateral liver plasma membrane, which was later proved to be identical to microsomal epoxide hydroxylase

[16]. On the other hand, Ananthanarayanan et al. reported the purification of a 49 kDa Na^+-dependent bile acid carrier from the rat basolateral liver plasma membrane [17]. However, there are uncertainties about the function of these proteins for Na^+-dependent bile acid uptake [15,17] and their physiological role remains to be proven.

Recently, Hagenbuch et al. reported the cloning and expression of an Na^+-dependent bile acid carrier at the basolateral liver plasma membrane in rats [18,19] and have postulated their secondary structure models [20]. The isolated protein has no significant homology to the 49 kDa or 49 kDa proteins mentioned above and its molecular weight is reported to be 51,000 [20]. The cloning of a human Na^+-dependent bile acid carrier at the basolateral liver plasma membrane has also been reported by the same group [21].

Although organic anions are taken up by hepatocytes by an Na^+-independent system [22–24], little is known about its relation to the Na^+-independent bile acid transport system. Furthermore, recent studies suggest an ATP-dependency for hepatic uptake of some organic anions [25,26].

Three different carriers have been reported for organic anion uptake at the basolateral liver plasma membrane [27–29]. These include two different proteins of 55 kDa (organic anion-binding protein [27] and BSP/bilirubin-binding protein [28]) and a 37 kDa protein called bilitranslocase [29].

Recently, Jacquemin et al. reported the expression of a basolateral Cl-dependent BSP carrier in Xenopus oocytes [30,31]. This protein had no significant homology to the organic anion carriers mentioned above [27–29]. The calculated molecular mass of this protein is 74 kDa and it also transports taurocholate and cholate [30,31], although its physiological importance in bile acid uptake remains to be elucidated.

Intracellular transport

Three different classes of cytosolic proteins which bind bile acids and organic anions in the rat and human liver have been reported [32–48]. Table 2 summarizes the binding affinities of rat and human hepatic binders for representative bile acids and organic anions. These proteins are considered to have an important role in the intracellular transport of ligands from the sinusoidal to the canalicular poles of the hepatocyte.

In the rat liver, Y protein (glutathione S-transferase) with a Y_a-subunit (ligandin) and Y′ protein have high binding affinity for bile acids. Amino acid conjugation decreases the binding affinity of these proteins for bile acids. Y and Z proteins have high affinity for organic anions. Rat Y′ protein is identical to 3α-hydroxysteroid dehydrogenase and has been shown to interact with bile acids in intact hepatocytes. Under physiological conditions, this protein acts as 3-oxoreductase of 3-oxo-bile acids produced by the intestinal bacteria.

Table 2. Binding affinities of bile acids and organic anions by cytosolic binders from rat and human liver

	Enzymatic activity	Molecular weight	Dissociation constant (μM)				
			Litho-cholate	Chenodeoxy-cholate	Cholate	Bilirubin	BSP
Rat							
Y protein	GST						
Y_aY_a		44,000	0.4	9	80	0.05	0.2
Y_bY_b		47,000	5	10	30	0.7	0.9
Y′ protein	3α-HSD	33,000	0.6	2	400	—	—
Z protein	—	14,000	5	80	700	0.3	0.7
Human							
Y protein	GST						
C_1		50,000	20	100	900	2.0	1.4
Y′ protein	DDH	36,000	0.03	0.08	2	—	—
Z protein	—	14,000	10	20	90	0.8	0.8

GST, glutathione S-transferase; 3α-HSD, 3α-hydroxysteroid dehydrogenase; DDH, dihydrodiol dehydrogenase. Data adapted from our previous reports [38–40,45].

In the human liver, Y′ protein has the highest binding affinity for bile acids. Different from the rat liver, human Y′ protein has only dihydrodiol dehydrogenase activity and 3α-hydroxysteroid dehydrogenases have been purified as different proteins with similar molecular weight [49]. Recently, the cloning and expression of rat and human Y′ bile acid binders have been reported and they have been shown to have high homologies to prostaglandin synthase [50,51]. Y and Z proteins also bind organic anions, but the binding affinity of human Y protein for organic anions is lower than that of rat Y protein with the Y_a-subunit (Table 2).

Vesicular transport of bile acids and organic anions has been postulated especially with their high-dose load [52–57]. The physiological importance of vesicular transport in the overall hepatic transport of bile acids and organic anions is unknown and studies against vesicular transport have recently been reported [58,59].

Canalicular excretion

The biliary excretion of bile acids has been reported to be mediated by electrogenic transport [60,61], and a 100 kDa protein was considered to be the electrogenic canalicular bile acid carrier [62,63]. However, an ATP-dependent bile acid carrier has been identified at the canalicular plasma membrane [64–66] and its molecular mass was reported to be 110 kDa [65]. Recently, Kast et al. found that the electrogenic bile acid carrier was due to the

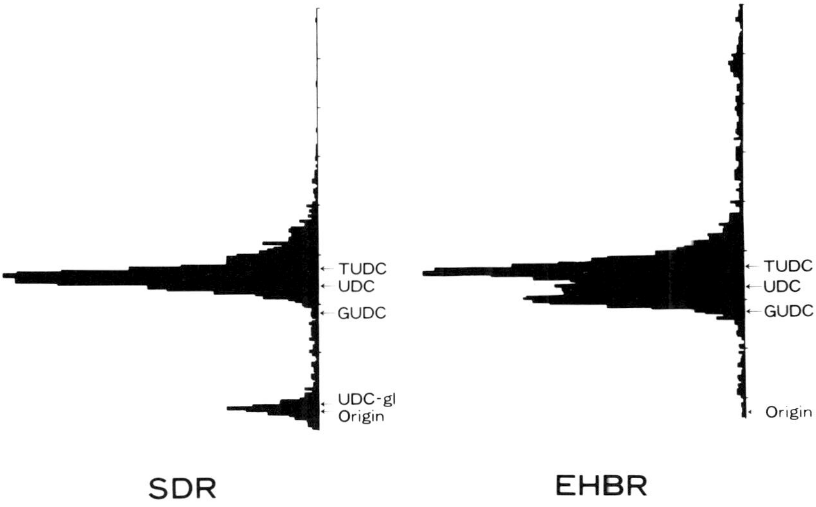

Fig. 5. The analyses of the bile samples after [^{14}C]ursodeoxycholate infusion at the rate of 1 μmol/min/100 b.wt. into a control Sprague-Dawley rat (SDR) and a hyperbilirubinemic mutant rat (EHBR) [72]. Aliquots of bile samples were analyzed by thin layer chromatography–radiochromatoscanner. The plate was developed by a solvent system of ethanol/ethyl acetate/ammonia (3/3/1, V/V) to separate glucuronides from other conjugates. UDC, ursodeoxycholate; TUDC, tauroursodeoxycholate; GUDC, glycoursodeoxycholate; UDC-gl, ursodeoxycholate-3-O-glucuronide.

contamination by microsomes of the canalicular plasma membrane vesicles used in the transport studies and that only the ATP-dependent carrier is localized at the canalicular membrane and has a role of bile acid excretion [67]. Although Wolters et al. reported the presence of ATP-dependent bile acid carriers at both the basolateral and canalicular plasma membrane of the human liver [68], the real localization of the ATP-dependent transporter awaits further studies due to the cross-contamination of the membrane marker enzymes in their liver plasma membrane preparations.

Mutant rats with conjugated hyperbilirubinemia have been reported; TR and GY rats of the Wistar strain [69,70] and Eisai hyperbilirubinemic rats (EHBRs) of the Sprague-Dawley strain [71]. In these mutant rats, a marked delay in biliary excretion of organic anions was observed, whereas biliary bile acid excretion was almost normal. Accordingly, an abnormal organic anion carrier at the canalicular plasma membrane has been considered to be the defect in these mutant rats [69–71]. The biliary excretion of bile acid glucuronides and sulfates is also impaired in these mutant rats. Figure 5 shows an analysis of the bile samples for the metabolites of intravenously administered ursodeoxycholate into rats. Ursodeoxycholate-3-O-glucuronide observed in the bile of a control Sprague-Dawley rat was not observed in the bile of EHBRs [72].

Thereafter, the existence of an ATP-dependent canalicular organic anion carrier has been reported and the ATP-dependent transport by canalicular plasma membrane vesicles of these mutant rats was defective [73–76]. However, two different groups exhibited opposite results for the mechanism of the transport of conjugated bilirubin, an important endogenous organic anion [77,78]. Further study is needed to resolve this controversy. Furthermore, Yi et al. reported the expression cloning of a putative rat canalicular reduced glutathione carrier [79], which may work as an organic anion carrier different from the ATP-dependent carrier at the canalicular plasma membrane. As reported by Sathirakul et al. [80], various lines of evidence support the view that there are more than two carriers for organic anions at the canalicular plasma membrane.

Hepatic transport of other compounds

Biliary excretion of cholesterol and phospholipids has been considered to be mediated by vesicular transport [81]. However, Berr et al. suggested the existence of a flippase for phospholipids at the canalicular plasma membrane, which transports phospholipids from the inside to the outside lipid bilayer of the canalicular plasma membrane [82]. Moreover, Smit et al. recently noted the absence of phospholipids in the bile of multidrug-resistance 2 gene knockout mice [83]. Their findings together with those reported by Cohen et al. [84], which suggest the importance of the phosphatidylcholine transfer protein in the intrahepatic transport of phospholipids, suggest that the phospholipid transport mechanism in the hepatocyte is different from the vesicular transport [81].

Intrahepatic transport of proteins is mediated by vesicular transport [85] and hepatic uptake of proteins is due either to a receptor-mediated or nonspecific endocytosis [86,87]. Recent reports by Hubbard and co-workers suggest that the canalicular plasma membrane proteins are first transported to the basolateral plasma membrane after synthesis, and then, to the canalicular plasma membrane [88,89].

Glutathione is synthesized in the liver and is subjected to carrier-mediated sinusoidal efflux or canalicular excretion [90,91]. Biliary excretion of organic cations such as anticancer drugs is mediated by P-glycoprotein, a multidrug-resistance gene product [92].

Cholestasis

Cholestasis is defined as a syndrome with decreased bile flow and regurgitation of biliary constituents such as bile acids, conjugated bilirubin and lipids into plasma. Figure 6 shows bile acid kinetics in cholestasis. Due to the

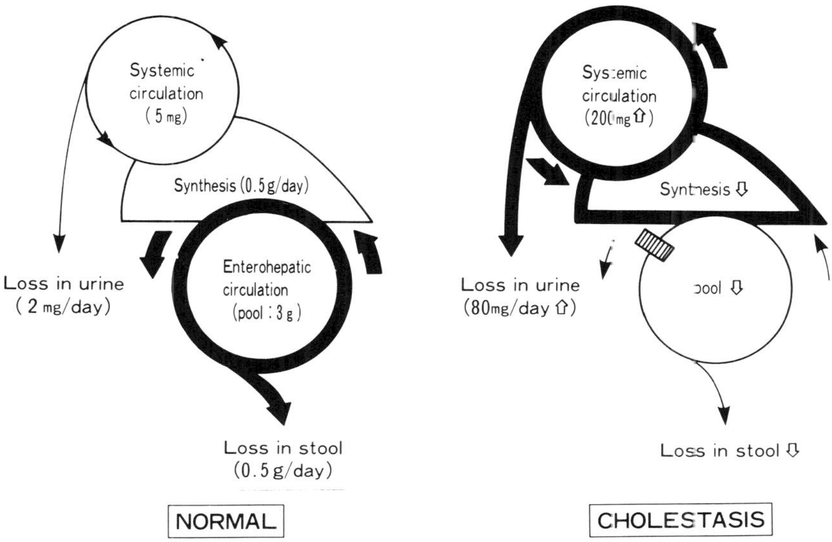

Fig. 6. Bile acid metabolism in normal subjects and in patients with cholestasis. Data in the schemas are mean values adopted from our previous reports [93–96].

Table 3. Experimental models for intrahepatic cholestasis

1. Hormones
   ethinylestradiol, estradiol-17β-glucuronide, norethandrolone
2. Microfilament inhibitors
   cytochalasin B, phalloidin
3. Drugs
   chlorpromazine, α-naphthylisothiocyanate, cyclosporine
4. Monohydroxy bile acids
   lithocholate, taurolithocholate, lithocholate-3-O-glucuronide
5. Others
   endotoxin, lymphokine

inhibition of the enterohepatic circulation, the bile acid pool moves to the systemic circulation and the liver, causing increases in serum bile acid levels and urinary bile acid excretion.

Although intrahepatic cholestasis is an important liver disease, its mechanisms are almost unknown. To study the pathogenesis of intrahepatic cholestasis, various experimental models have been used [1–4], which include hormones, microfilament inhibitors, some drugs, and monohydroxy bile acids (Table 3).

Several mechanisms have been postulated for various experimental models of intrahepatic cholestasis (Fig. 7): 1) Inhibition of Na,K-ATPase and 2)

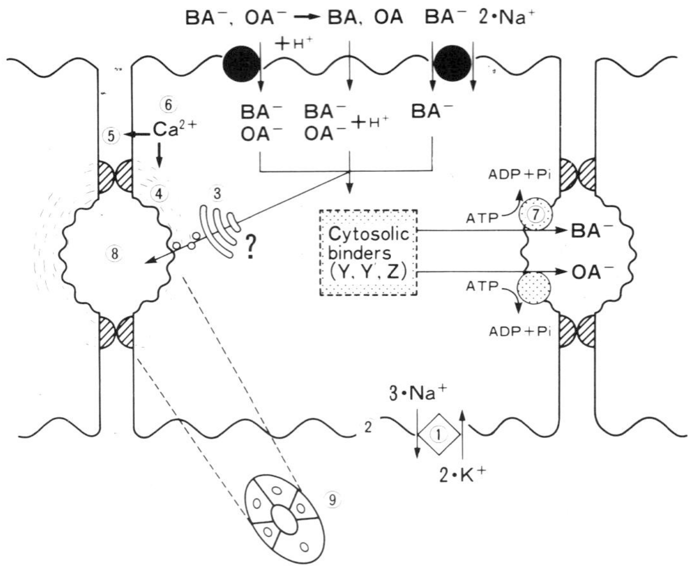

Fig. 7. Mechanisms of intrahepatic cholestasis. See the text for the explanation of the numbers (1–9) in the figure.

altered fluidity of the basolateral plasma membrane, causing the inhibition of bile acid uptake, cytoskeletal alterations such as 3) microtubule dysfunction to decrease the intrahepatic vesicular transport or 4) microfilament dysfunction to decrease the canalicular contraction, 5) increased permeability of the tight junction, 6) increased cytosolic Ca^{2+}, which also affects microfilament function and the permeability of the tight junction, 7) a decrease in the numbers of the canalicular bile acid carrier, 8) precipitation of cholestatic compounds in the bile canaliculi, and 9) damages to the intrahepatic bile duct. However, little is known concerning which mechanism is essential for each experimental model [1–4].

Ethinylestradiol-induced cholestasis

Among various experimental models, ethinylestradiol-induced cholestasis is the most frequently used, since estrogen is considered to be a cause of benign recurrent cholestasis in pregnancy. The intramuscular administration of ethinylestradiol for several days to rats causes cholestasis. As mechanisms of estrogen-induced cholestasis, an increased permeability of the tight junction [97,98], and an altered fluidity of the basolateral plasma membrane and inhibition of Na,K-ATPase which inhibit the Na^+-dependent bile acid uptake

[99–101] have been posulated. However, later studies revealed that the permeability of the tight junction does not change [102] or that cholestasis precedes the permeability change [103] in estrogen-induced cholestasis. Furthermore, findings against the importance of the membrane fluidity and Na,K-ATPase in estrogen-induced cholestasis have been reported; Na-independent organic anion uptake is also impaired, cholestasis precedes the changes of Na,K-ATPase and membrane fluidity [104], and spironolactone decreases membrane fluidity whereas it increases bile flow [105]. According to these reports, although increased permeability of the tight junction, decreased membrane fluidity and the inhibition of Na,K-ATPase are observed in estrogen-induced cholestasis, they do not seem to be involved in the initiation of cholestasis.

Recent reports suggest that estrogens bind to the estrogen receptor and change the synthesis of carrier proteins or actin, or that estrogen metabolites cause cholestasis [106,107]. Estradiol-17β-glucuronide is known to cause cholestasis in rats [108,109]. Romaneli et al. reported that ethinylestradiol treatment inhibits the ATP-dependent canalicular bile acid transport, suggesting a decrease in the number of canalicular bile acid carriers (Fig. 7) [110]. However, further studies are needed to determine the fundamental mechanism of estrogen-induced cholestasis.

Lithocholate-3-O-glucuronide-induced cholestasis

Lithocholate, a monohydroxy bile acid, has been reported to cause cholestasis in rats. Oelberg et al. first reported that a glucuronide of lithocholate, lithocholate-3-O-glucuronide, is also a cholestatic agent [111].

Figure 8 shows the effects of lithocholate and its conjugates on bile flow in rats. Lithocholate-3-O-glucuronide was more cholestatic than lithocholate whereas lithocholate-3-sulfate did not change bile flow at the same dose [112]. Since the cytotoxic effect of lithocholate-3-O-glucuronide on isolated rat hepatocytes was lower than that of lithocholate [14], different mechanisms other than hepatotoxicity may be working in lithocholate-3-O-glucuronide-induced cholestasis. Electron microscopic studies revealed only minor histological changes in lithocholate-3-O-glucuronide-induced cholestasis [113], which is in contrast to that in taurolithocholate-induced cholestasis; dilatation and a typical lamellar transformation of the canalicular plasma membrane [114]. In EHBRs, in which biliary lithocholate-3-O-glucuronide excretion is markedly impaired [114], a cholestatic dose of lithocholate-3-O-glucuronide to control rats (0.1 μmol/min/100 g b.wt. for 40 min) failed to induce cholestasis [115]. These findings indicate that biliary excretion of lithocholate-3-O-glucuronide is needed to cause cholestasis. However, in comparing the cholestatic effect of different lithocholate-3-O-glucuronide doses (0.1 versus

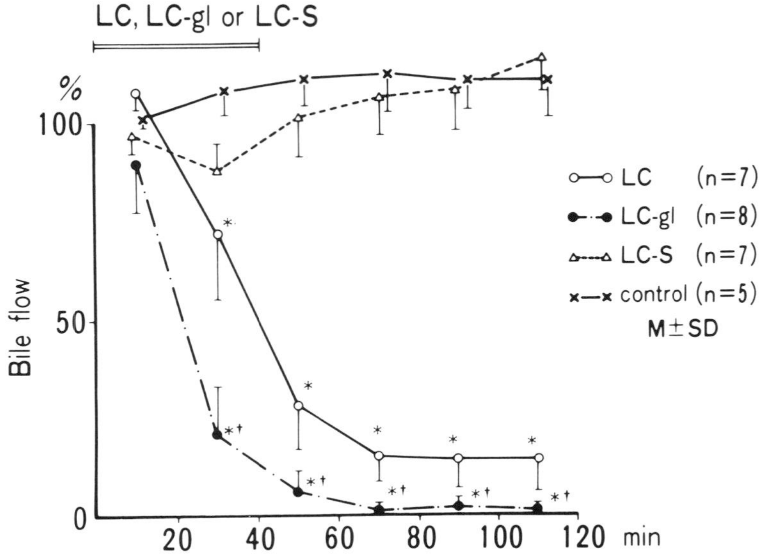

Fig. 8. Effects of lithocholate and its conjugates on bile flow. Bile acids were intravenously administered to rats at the rate of 0.29 μmol/min/100 g b.wt. for 40 min [112]. LC, lithocholate; LC-gl, lithocholate-3-O-glucuronide; LC-S, lithocholate-3-sulfate.

0.3 μmol/min/100 g b.wt. for 40 min), biliary concentrations of lithocholate-3-O-glucuronide did not correlate to the severity of cholestasis. These findings suggest that cholestasis occurs before or during the transport of lithocholate-3-O-glucuronide through the canalicular plasma membrane [115].

Figure 9 shows the effect of lithocholate-3-O-glucuronide on biliary glutathione excretion, which may contribute to the bile acid-independent canalicular bile flow. A low dose of lithocholate-3-O-glucuronide (1.6 μmol/100 g b.wt.), causing moderate cholestasis, markedly inhibited biliary glutathione excretion, indicating that the inhibition of bile acid-independent canalicular bile flow is the first step in 3-glcA-LC-induced cholestasis [116].

We recently reported that the treatment with colchicine, a vesicular transport inhibitor, inhibited lithocholate-3-O-glucuronide-induced cholestasis [117]. This was not observed in lumicolchicine-treated rats, while pretreatment with vinblastine, another vesicular transport inhibitor, also inhibited lithocholate-3-O-glucuronide-induced cholestasis. These findings indicate that the intrahepatic transport of lithocholate-3-O-glucuronide by the vesicular pathway may cause cholestasis [113,117]. However, further studies are needed to fully determine the pathogenesis of lithocholate-3-O-glucuronide-induced cholestasis.

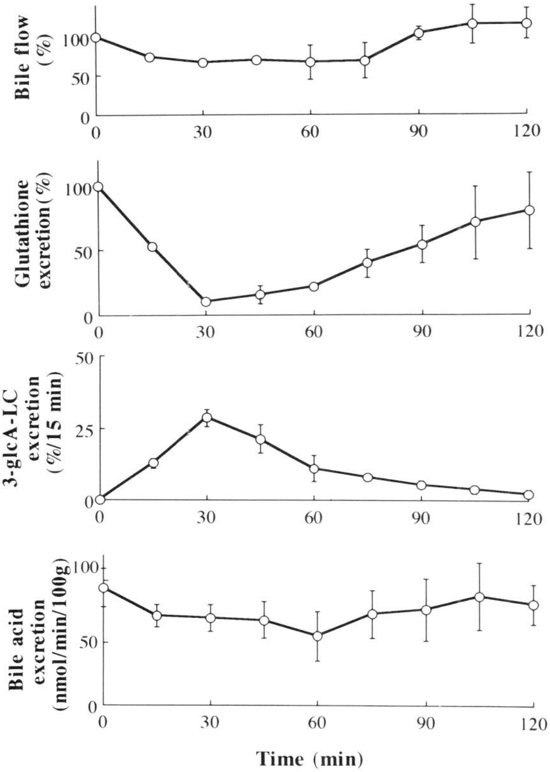

Fig. 9. Effect of lithocholate-3-O-glucuronide (3-glcA-LC) on biliary glutathione excretion [115]. ^{14}C-labeled 3-glcA-LC (1.6 μmol/100 g b.wt.) was intravenously administered to rats and bile samples were collected every 15 min.

References

1. Reichen J, Simon FR, Cholestasis. In: Arias IM, Jacoby WB, Popper H et al. (eds) The liver biology and pathobiology. 2nd Edition. New York: Raven Press, 1988;1105–1124.
2. Scharschmidt BF. Bile formation and cholestasis. In: Zakim D, Boyer TD (eds) Hepatology. A text book of liver disease. 2nd Edition. Philadelphia: WB Saunders, 1990;303–340.
3. Reichen J. Mechanisms of cholestasis. In: Tavoloni N, Berk PD (eds) Hepatic transport and bile secretion. Physiology and pathophysiology. New York: Raven Press, 1993;665–672.
4. Fallon MB, Anderson JM, Boyer JL. Intrahepatic cholestasis. In: Schiff L, Schiff ER (eds) Diseases of the liver. 7th Edition. Philadelphia: JB Lippincott, 1993;343–361.
5. Ballatori N, Truong AT. Am J Physiol 1992;263:G22–G30.
6. Ballatori N, Truong AT. Am J Physiol 1992;263:G617–G624.
7. Reichen J, Paumgartner G. Am J Physiol 1976;231:734–742.
8. Anwer MS, Hedner D. Hoppe-Seyler's Z Physiol Chem 1978;359:181–192.
9. van Dyke RW, Stephans JE, Scharschmidt BF. Am J Physiol 1982;243:484–492.

10. Takikawa H, Takemura T, Yamanaka M. Int Hepatol Commun 1995;3:20–25.
11. Inoue M, Kinne R, Tran T et al. Hepatology 1982;2:572–579.
12. Zimmerli B, Valantinas J, Meier P. J Pharmacol Exp Ther 1989;250:301–308.
13. Blitzer BL, Terzakis C, Scott KA. J Biol Chem 1986;261:12042–12046.
14. Takikawa H, Tomita J, Takemura T et al. Biochim Biophys Acta 1991;1091:173–178.
15. von Dippe P, Levy D. J Biol Chem 1990;263:14812–14816.
16. Alves CH, von Dippe P, Amoni M et al. J Biol Chem 1993;268:20148–20155.
17. Ananthanarayanan M, Bucuvalas JC, Schneider BL et al. Am J Physiol 1991;261:G810–G817.
18. Hagenbuch B, Lübbert H, Stieger B et al. J Biol Chem 1990;265:5357–5360.
19. Hagenbuch B, Stieger B, Foguet M et al. Proc Natl Acad Sci USA 1991;88:10629–10633.
20. Meier PJ, Hagenbuch B, Stieger B et al. In: Keppler D, Jungermann K (eds) Transport in the liver. Dordrecht: Kluwer, 1994;38–48.
21. Hagenbuch B, Meier PJ. J Clin Invest 1994;93:1326–1331.
22. Scharschmidt BF, Waggoner JG, Berk PD. J Clin Invest 1975;56:1280–1292.
23. Schwenk M, Burr R, Schwarz L et al. Eur J Biochem 1976;64:189–197.
24. Schwenk M. Arch Toxicol 1980;44:113–126.
25. Yamazaki M, Suzuki H, Sugiyama Y et al. J Hepatol 1992;14:41–47.
26. Yamazaki M, Suzuki H, Hanano M et al. Am J Physiol 1993;264:G693–G701.
27. Wolkoff AW, Chung CT. J Clin Invest 1980;65:1152–1161.
28. Berk PD, Potter BJ, Stemmel W. Hepatology 1987;7:1326–1331.
29. Tiribelli C, Lunazzi GC, Sottocasa GL. Biochim Biophys Acta 1990;1031:261–275.
30. Jacquemin E, Hagenbuch B, Stieger B et al. J. Clin Invest 1991;88:2146–2149.
31. Jacquemin E, Hagenbuch B, Stieger B et al. Proc Natl Acad Sci USA 1994;91:133–137.
32. Levy AJ, Gatmaitan Z, Arias IM. J Clin Invest 1969;48:2156–2169.
33. Wolkoff AF, Goresky CA, Sellin J et al. Am J Physiol 1979;236:E638–E648.
34. Sugiyama Y, Yamada T, Kaplowitz N. J Biol Chem 1983;258:3602–3607.
35. Sugiyama Y, Sugimoto M, Stolz A et al. Biochem Pharmacol 1984;33:3511–3513.
36. Stolz A, Sugiyama Y, Kuhlenkamp J et al. FEBS Lett 1984;177:31–35.
37. Takikawa H, Sugiyama Y, Stolz A et al. Biochem Pharmacol 1986;35:343–346.
38. Takikawa H, Stolz A, Sugimoto M et al. J Lipid Res 1986;27:652–657.
39. Takikawa H, Sugiyama Y, Kaplowitz N. J Lipid Res 1986;27:955–966.
40. Takikawa H, Kaplowitz N. Arch Biochem Biophys 1986;251:385–392.
41. Stolz A, Takikawa H, Sugiyama Y et al. J Clin Invest 1987;79:427–434.
42. Takikawa H, Stolz A, Kaplowitz N. J Clin Invest 1987;80:852–860.
43. Takikawa H, Ookhtens M, Stolz A et al. J Clin Invest 1987;80:861–866.
44. Takikawa H, Kaplowitz N. J Lipid Res 1988;29:279–286.
45. Takikawa H, Sugiyama Y, Kaplowitz N. Biochim Biophys Acta 1988;954:37–43.
46. Takikawa H, Stolz A, Sugiyama Y et al. J Biol Chem 1990;265:2132–2136.
47. Takikawa H, Stolz A, Kuroki S et al. Biochim Biophys Acta 1990;1043:153–156.
48. Takikawa H, Fernandez-Checa JC, Kuhlenkamp J et al. Biochim Biophys Acta 1991;1084:247–250.
49. Takikawa H, Fujiyoshi H, Nishikawa K et al. Hepatology 1992;16:365–371.
50. Stolz A, Rahimi-Kiani M, Ameis D et al. J Biol Chem 1991;266:15253–15257.
51. Stolz A, Hammand J, Lou H et al. J Biol Chem 1993;268:10448–10457.
52. Suchy FJ, Balistreri WF, Hung J et al. Am J Physiol 1983;245:G681–G689.
53. Mori M, Oyamada M, Sakauchi F et al. Virchows Arch B 1987;53:37–43.
54. Crawford JM, Gollan JL. Am J Physiol 1988;255:G121–G131.
55. Lamri Y, Roda A, Dumont M et al. J Clin Invest 1988;82:1173–1182.
56. Kitamura T, Gatmaitan Z, Arias IM. Hepatology 1990; 12:1358–1364.
57. Dumont M, D'Hont C, Durand-Schneider A-M et al. Hepatology 1991;14:10–15.
58. Reynier MO, Hashieh IA, Crotte C et al.Gastroenterology 1992;102:2024–2032.

59. Crawford JM, Barnes S, Stearns RC et al. Lab Invest 1994;71:42–51.
60. Inoue M, Kinne R, Tran T et al. J Clin Invest 1984;73:659–663.
61. Meier PJ, Meier-Abt AS, Barnett C et al. J Biol Chem 1984;259:10614–10622.
62. Ruetz S, Fricker G, Hugentobler G et al. J Biol Chem 1987;62:11324–11330.
63. Sippel CJ, Ananthanarayanan M, Suchy FJ. Am J Physiol 1990;258:G728–G737.
64. Adachi Y, Kobayashi H, Kurumi Y et al. Hepatology 1991;14:655–659.
65. Müller M, Ishikawa T, Berger U et al. J Biol Chem 1991;266:18920–18926.
66. Nishida T, Gatmaitan Z, Che M et al. Proc Natl Acad Sci USA 1991;88:6590–6594.
67. Kast C, Stieger B, Winteerhalter KH et al. J Biol Chem 1994;269:5179–5186.
68. Wolters H, Kuipers F, Slooff MJH et al. J Clin Invest 1922;90:2321–2326.
69. Jansen PLM, Peters WH, Lamers WH. Hepatology 1985;4:573–579.
70. Kuipers F, Enserink M, Havinga R et al. J Clin Invest 1988;81:1593–1599.
71. Takikawa H, Sano N, Narita T et al. Hepatology 1991;14:352–360.
72. Takikawa H, Sano N, Minagawa K et al. J Hepatol 1992;15:77–84.
73. Kobayashi K, Sogame Y, Hara H et al. J Biol Chem 1990;265:7737–7741.
74. Ishikawa T, Müller M, Klünemann C et al. J Biol Chem 1990;265:19279–19286.
75. Kitamura T, Jansen P, Hardenbrook C et al. Proc Natl Acad Sci USA 1990;87:7737–7741.
76. Fernandez-Checa JC, Takikawa H, Horie T et al. J Biol Chem 1991;267:1667–1673.
77. Adachi Y, Kobayashi H, Kurumi Y et al. Hepatology 1991;14:1251–1258.
78. Nishida T, Gatmaitan Z, Roy-Chawdhry J et al. J Clin Invest 1992;90:2130–2135.
79. Yi J-R, Lu S, Fernandez-Checa J et al. J Clin Invest 1994;93:1841–1845.
80. Sathirakul K, Suzuki H, Yasuda K et al J Pharmacol Exp Ther 1993;265:1301–1312.
81. Coleman R, Rahman K, Bellringer ME et al. In: Northfield T, Jazrawi R, Zentler-Munro P (eds) Bile acids in health and disease. Dordrecht: Kluwer, 1988;43–60.
82. Berr E, Meier PJ, Stieger B. J Biol Chem 1993;268:1–4.
83. Smit JJM, Schinkel AH, Oude Elferink RPJ et al. Cell 1993;75:451–462.
84. Cohen DE, Leonard MR, Carey MC. Biochemistry 1994;33:9975–9980.
85. Renston RH, Maloney DG, Jones AL et al. Gastroenterology 1980;78:1373–1388.
86. Bridges K, Harford J, Ashwell G et al. Proc Natl Acad Sci USA 1982;79:350–354.
87. Sato H, Sugiyama Y, Sawada Y et al. Am J Physiol 1990;258:G682–G689.
88. Bartles JR, Feracci HM, Stieger B et al J Cell Biol 1987;105:1241–1251.
89. Maurice M, Schell MJ, Lardeux B et al. Hepatology 1994;19:648–655.
90. Ookhtens M, Hobdy K, Corvasce MC et al. J Clin Invest 1985;75:258–265.
91. Fernandez-Checa JC, Ookhtens M, Kaplowitz N. J Biol Chem 1993;268:10836–10841.
92. Kamimoto Y, Gatmaitan Z, Hsu et al. J Biol Chem 1989;264:11693–11698.
93. Takikawa H, Otsuka H, Beppu T et al. J Biochem 1982;92:985–998.
94. Takikawa H, Otsuka H, Beppu T et al. Digestion 1983;27:189–195.
95. Takikawa H, Beppu T, Seyama Y. Gastroenterol Jpn 1984;19:104–109.
96. Takikawa H, Otsuka H, Beppu T et al. Biochem Med 1985;33:393–400.
97. Forker EL. J Clin Invest 1964;48:654–663.
98. Robenek H, Rassat J, Grosser V et al. Virchows Arch Cell Pathol 1982;40:201–215.
99. Davis RA, Kera F, Showalter R et al. Proc Natl Acad Sci USA 1978;75:4130–4134.
100. Keeffe EB, Scharschmidt BR, Blankenship NM et al. J Clin Invest 1979;64:1590–1598.
101. Berr F, Simon FR, Reichen J. Am J Physiol 1984;247:G437–G443.
102. Jaeschke H, Krell H, Pfaff E. Gastroenterology 1983;85:808–814.
103. Jaeschke H, Trummer E, Krell H. Gastroenterology 1987;93:533–538.
104. Boelsterli UA, Rakhit G, Balazs T. Hepatology 1983;3:12–17.
105. Smith DJ, Gordon ER. J. Lab Clin Med 1988;112:679–685.
106. Vore M. Gastroenterology 1987;993:643–649.
107. Reyes-Romero MA. Medical Hypotheses 1990;32:39–43.
108. Meyers M, Slikker W, Pascoe G et al. J Pharmacol Exp Ther 1980;214:87–93.
109. Sano N, Takikawa H, Yamanaka M. J Hepatol 1993;17:241–246.

110. Bossard R, Stieger B, O'Neill B et al. J Clin Invest 1993;91:2714–2720.
111. Oelberg DG, Chari MV, Little JM et al. J Clin Invest 1984;73:1507–1514.
112. Takikawa H, Ohki H, Sano N et al. Biochim Biophys Acta 1991;1081:39–44.
113. Takikawa H, Sano N, Wako Y et al. In: Keppler D, Jungemann K (eds) Transport in the liver. Kluwer: Dordrecht, 1994;192–199.
114. Miyai K, Mayr WW, Richardson AL. Lab Invest 1975;32:527–535.
115. Takikawa H, Minagawa K, Sano N et al. Dig Dis Sci 1993;38:1543–1548.
116. Takikawa H, Sano N, Yamazaki R et al. Int Hepatol Commun 1995;3:48–52.
117. Takikawa H, Sano N, Yamazaki R et al. J Hepatol 1995;22:88–93.

Progress in Hepatology Vol. 1.
Cellular and Molecular Biology.
M. Yamanaka, K. Okabe and G. Toda, editors.

Hepatocyte growth factor: pleiotrophic roles for liver regeneration and possible clinical applications

Hisashi Amaike, Kunio Matsumoto, and Toshikazu Nakamura
Division of Biochemistry, Department of Oncology, Biomedical Research Center, Osaka University, Medical School, Suita, Osaka 565, Japan

Abstract. Hepatocyte growth factor (HGF), originally identified in sera of partially hepatectomized rats as a novel growth factor for mature hepatocytes, is a heterodimeric molecule composed of a 69 kD α-subunit and a 34 kD of β-subunit. HGF is produced by mesenchymal or stromal cells and acts on a wide variety of epithelial cells and endothelial cells as mitogen, motogen, and morphogen. In an animal model of liver ischemia or hepatitis, rapid induction of HGF mRNA occurs in the injured liver and HGF produced in nonparenchymal liver cells acts on injured parenchymal hepatocytes through a paracrine mechanism. On the other hand, HGF derived from the blood circulation triggers liver regeneration in case of partial hepatectomy as a rapid induction of HGF expression occurs in distal, intact organs. Moreover, HGF acts as a "trophic factor" for regeneration of kidneys and lungs. Administration of recombinant HGF into experimental animals accelerates the regeneration of the liver and kidney and prevents the onset of severe acute organ failure. HGF is now considered to be a pleiotropic factor which regulates cell growth, angiogenesis and tissue construction during embryogenesis, organogenesis, and organ regeneration, through unique biological activities.

Key words: acute renal failure, *c-MET*/HGF receptor, HGF, injurin, liver cirrhosis, organotrophic factor.

Introduction

Hepatocyte growth factor (HGF) is a cytokine and a most potent hepatotrophic factor for liver regeneration [1–4]. In the plasma of partially hepatectomized rats, we found a humoral factor which stimulated DNA synthesis of rat mature hepatocytes in primary culture. We named it "HGF" [1], and purified HGF from a large amount of rat platelets [5,6].

In 1989 and 1990, both rat and human HGF cDNA were molecularly cloned and primary structures were determined [7–10]. HGF was also purified from human plasma [11,12] and the conditioned medium of human lung fibroblasts [13]. HGF has been shown to act as mitogen (stimulation of cell

Address for correspondence: Dr Toshikazu Nakamura, Division of Biochemistry, Department of Oncology, Biomedical Research Center, Osaka University Medical School, Suita, Osaka 565, Japan. Fax: 81-6-879-3789.

proliferation), motogen (stimulation of cell motility), and morphogen (induction of tissue structure) for various types of cells [14–18]. Moreover, HGF elicits "trophic function" for regeneration of many organs, including the lung and the kidney, as well as the liver [4,17–22].

HGF is thus considered to be a pleiotropic factor which regulates not only cell growth but also the tissue construction during embryogenesis, organogenesis, and organ regeneration [17,18]. HGF has attracted much attention from researchers of cancer [23–27], developmental biology [28–30], and clinically in hepatology [31], nephrology [32], respiratology [22], hematology [33,34], and orthopedics [35].

Biochemical characteristics of HGF

HGF is a disulfide-linked heterodimeric molecule composed of a 69 kD α-subunit and a 34 kD β-subunit [5,6,11,12]. HGF is a heat- and acid-labile protein. Biological activities are lost by boiling for 1.5 min, treatment with 1 M acetic acid, trypsin digestion, and reduction with dithiothreitol [5]. The amino acids sequence of rat HGF is 91% identical with that of human HGF, indicating that the primary structure of HGF is highly conserved among species [7,9]. HGF has no species specificity in biological activity between human and Xenopus.

The *c-met* was originally isolated as a transforming gene from a human osteogenic sarcoma cell line transformed with the chemical carcinogen N-methyl-N′-nitro-N-nitrosoguanidine in 1984 [36]. This proto-oncogene product (*c-MET*) was found to be a specific receptor for HGF [37–39]. *c-MET* is composed of a 50 kD α-subunit and a 145 kD β-subunit of transmembrane tyrosine kinase [38,40] and the biological activities of HGF are specifically expressed after binding to the receptor [18,39,41,42]. This high-affinity *c-MET*/HGF receptor with a Kd value of 20–30 pM is widely distributed in various tissues and is expressed 100–1,500 sites/cell on the plasma membrane [43–45]. On the other hand, HGF has strong affinity for heparin [1,5,6,11,12,46] and also binds to the heparan sulfate in the extracellular matrix in vivo [47,48]. Heparan sulfate on the cell surface and extracellular matrix is thought to act as the reservoir of HGF in vivo, on the basis of pharmacokinetical studies for the clearance of human recombinant HGF (hr-HGF) injected into experimental animals [49].

HGF has one N-terminal hairpin loop domain and four kringle domains. Kringle domains are found in proteases involved in blood-coagulation and in fibrinolysis pathways. Studies using variously mutated recombinant HGFs revealed that the N-terminal hairpin-loop domain and the first or second kringle domain are essential for the binding of HGF to *c-MET*/HGF receptor [50] and various biological activities are lost when these domains are deleted [51]. The β-subunit has a serine protease-like structure and has 37%

homology in amino acid sequence to plasminogen. However, HGF has no proteolytic activity because two amino acids in the active triad, Serine and Histidine, are replaced by Tyrosine and Glutamine in HGF, respectively [7].

Expression of HGF gene

The HGF gene is mapped on q21.1 of chromosome 7 in humans [52]. It is composed of 18 exons interrupted with 17 introns, and is about 70 kb long [53]. Single stranded prepro-HGF composed of 728 amino acids is initially translated from 6 kb mRNA, and 31 amino acids of N-terminal signal sequence are cleaved before secretion of HGF. Subsequently, pro-HGF is cleaved between Arg^{494} and Val^{495} extracellularly, resulting in the formation of a biologically active two-chain mature HGF [7,54,55]. This processing pathway and structure of the mature form of HGF are schematically described in Fig. 1.

Activation of HGF from the single to chain HGF is catalyzed by a specific serine protease, "HGF-converting enzyme" [54]. This recently purified enzyme proved to be a heterodimeric molecule composed of a 65 kD subunit and a 32 kD subunit. Since the catalytic activity is nine times higher in the serum than in the plasma, tissue injury and the concomitant blood coagulation reactions may be responsible for its activation. Shimomura et al. [55] also purified a serine protease with similar catalytic properties, termed "HGF activator". But the molecular weight of "HGF activator" purified from human serum (34 kD protein composed of 30 kD and 4 kD) differs from that of "HGF converting enzyme". The catalytic domain of HGF activator has 47% homology to the blood coagulation factor XII [56]. The factor XII is cleaved to two isoforms, α-XIIa consisting of two subunits of 52 kD and 28 kD or β-XIIb consisting of 2 kD and 28 kD subunits, by limited proteolysis. Similar proteolytic processing in factor XII may exist in the activation of precursor of HGF-processing enzyme and cause the difference in the size between "HGF converting enzyme" and "HGF activator", further structural analysis in these enzymes is needed to elucidate the relation between "HGF converting enzyme" and "HGF activator".

Pleiotrophic activities of HGF

Epidermal growth factor (EGF) and transforming growth factor-α (TGF-α) are also potent growth factors for hepatocytes, however, even 0.5 ng/ml (6 pM) of HGF stimulates the DNA synthesis of hepatocytes and the maximum mitogenic activity is 2–3 fold stronger than that of EGF or TGF-α, i.e., HGF is heretofore the most potent mitogen for hepatocytes [5,6]. HGF was initially described as a hepatocyte-specific growth factor, but it is now

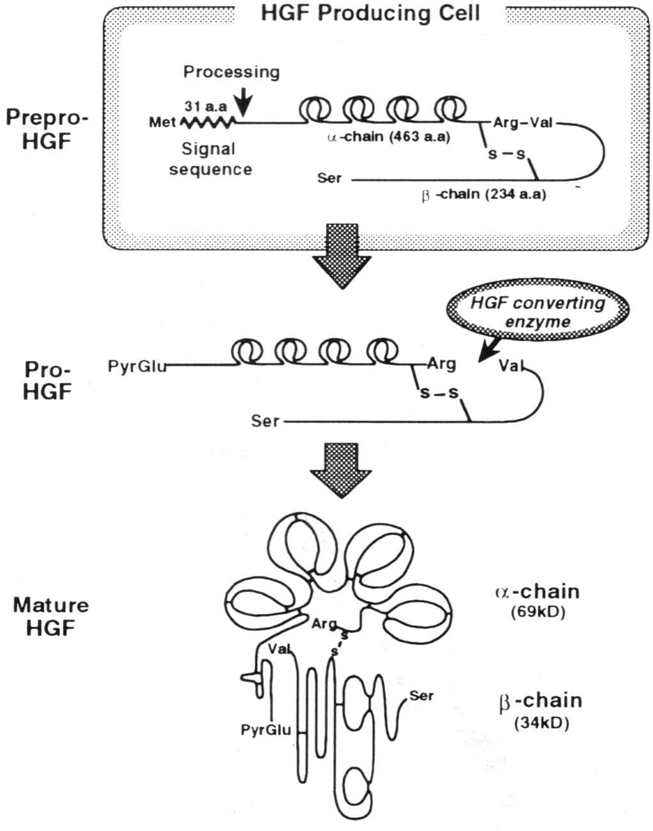

Fig. 1. Schematic presentation of the processing of HGF and structure of mature HGF.

considered to be a pleiotropic factor which targets a wide variety of cells. As shown in Table 1, HGF is a potent mitogen predominantly for epithelial cells, such as human keratinocytes [57], melanocytes [17], renal tubular epithelial cells [58], bronchial epithelial cells, alveolar type II epithelial cells [59], and pancreatic aciner cells. Recent studies have shown that HGF also stimulates the growth of some kinds of cells derived from mesenchymal tissue, such as vascular endothelial cells [60,61], and hematopoietic progenitor cells [33,34].

A scatter factor which stimulates epithelial cell motility was identified as the same molecule as HGF in 1991 [41,62,63]. HGF elicits motogenic activity for various types of epithelial cells. Moreover, Montesano et al. [14] and Johonson et al. [64] showed that HGF induced a branching tubular structure in MDCK renal tubular epithelial cells and hepatic bile duct epithelial cells, acting as an epithelial morphogen.

In contrast to the mitogenic action of HGF for the normal epithelium, HGF

Table 1. Biological characteristics of HGF

Maximum activity	5~10 ng/ml (60~80 pM)
Metabolic action	Stimulation of albumin synthesis (hepatocyte)
	Stimulation of Na^+-K^+ATPase (renal tubular epithelium)
Additivity of effect	With EGF, TGF-α, and insulin
Species specificity	None known
Target cells	
Growth stimulation	Hepatocyte
	Human keratinocyte
	Bronchial epithelium
	Thyroid follicular epithelium
	Renal tubular epithelium
	Human melanocyte
	Alveolar type II cell
	Pancreatic acinar cell
Growth inhibition	Hep G2 (human hepatoma)
	KB (human squamous cell carcinoma)
	B6/F1 (mouse melanoma) etc.
Morphogenic activity	MDCK (canine renal tubular epithelium)
	Bile duct epithelium
	Mammary gland epithelium etc.
Motogenic activity	Human keratinocyte
	Oral mucosal epithelium
	A431 (human epidermoid carcinoma)
	Gall bladder epithelium
	MDCK
	Hep G2

suppresses the growth of cancer cells [24], as shown in Table 1. Shiota et al [27] showed that the tumor-inhibitory effect of HGF on hepatocellular carcinoma cells is functional in nude mice in vivo: the tumorigenicity and tumor size of hepatoma cells were much decreased when the cells were transfected with the expression vector for HGF. Furthermore, tumor cytotoxic factor (F-TCF) purified from conditioned medium of human lung embryonic fibroblasts was shown to be an identical molecule to HGF [25,26].

As mentioned above, HGF has the various kinds of biological activities, predominantly for a wide variety of epithelial cells. Based on these multipotent actions, HGF is now considered to be a pleiotropic factor which plays important roles in the regeneration of adult organs such as liver, kidney, and lung, as well as in epithelial-mesenchymal interactions during organogenesis.

HGF as a hepatotrophic factor for liver regeneration

Blood levels of HGF are rapidly elevated after liver injuries caused by hepatotoxins such as carbon tetrachloride (CCl_4) and D-galactosamine [19],

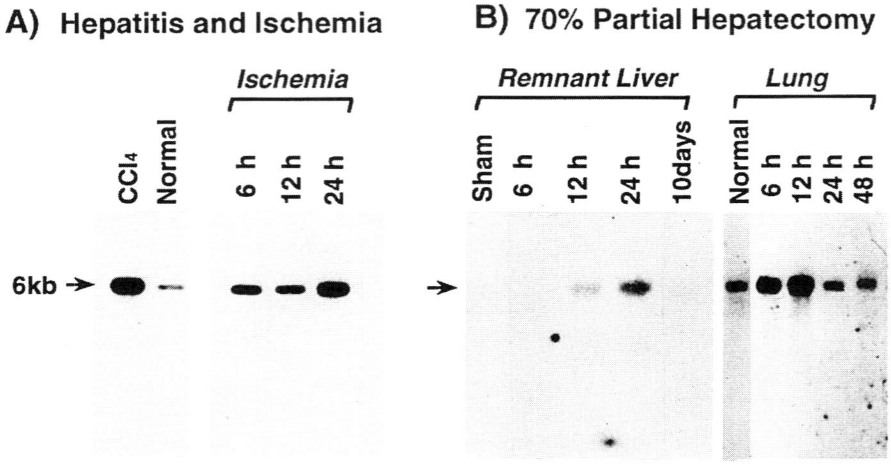

Fig. 2. Induction of HGF mRNA in rat liver with various types of injury. A: Changes in the liver after CCl_4 administration or ischemia. B: Changes in the remnant liver or intact lung after 70% partial hepatectomy.

ischemia with partial ligation of the portal vein [65], and partial hepatectomy [66,67] in rats. Our experiments indicate that HGF acts on liver regeneration, in an endocrine and/or paracrine fashion as follows:

Paracrine mechanism of HGF action

When acute and severe cellular damage to hepatocytes is caused by the ingestion of CCl_4 or by liver ischemia, HGF mRNA expression in the liver increases remarkably within a few hours and reaches a maximal level after 10–24 hours [19] (Fig. 2A). Blood HGF levels are also increased several hours later and DNA synthesis of hepatocytes reaches a peak at 24–48 hours after the treatment. HGF mRNA was specifically expressed in the non-parenchymal liver cells [19], such as Kupffer cells, hepatic sinusoidal endothelial cells [68], and Ito cells [69,70], as detected by Northern blot hybridization and in situ hybridization. On the other hand, the expression of HGF mRNA in distal intact organs such as lung and spleen is not so remarkably enhanced in such cases. Therefore, HGF derived from non-parenchymal cells in a paracrine fashion may stimulate the proliferation of hepatocytes when these tissues are subjected to insult.

Endocrine mechanism of HGF action

In the case of 70% partial hepatectomy in rats, as shown in Figure 2B, HGF mRNA expression in the remnant liver increased from 12 hours and reached a

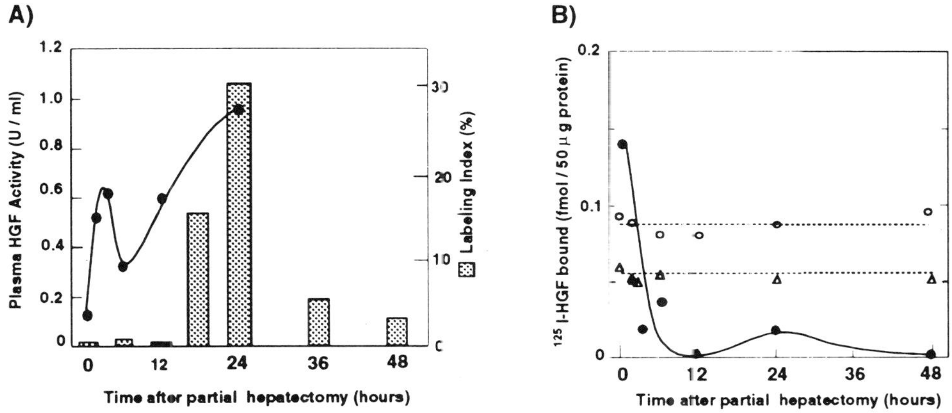

Fig. 3. Changes in HGF activity in the plasma, DNA synthesis in hepatocytes, and expression of *c-MET*/HGF receptor in rats after 70% partial hepatectomy. A: HGF activity in the plasma (●) and DNA synthesis in hepatocytes (▩) of 70% hepatectomized rat. HGF activity was determined by measuring DNA synthesis of adult rat hepatocytes in primary culture. DNA synthesis in the remnant liver was determined by BrdU incorporation into hepatocytes. B: Specific binding of ^{125}I-HGF to plasma membranes of liver, kidney, and lung, after 70% partial hepatectomy: ●, liver; ○, kidney; △, lung.

maximum after 24 hours after surgery [66]. However, the increase of HGF mRNA expression in the remnant liver was much less and later than that in the case of CCl_4 administration. On the other hand, the level of expression of HGF mRNA in the intact lung increased 5-fold at 6 hours and was about 20-fold higher at 12 hours after hepatectomy [71]. This rapid induction of HGF mRNA was seen in lung, spleen, and kidney [72]. HGF induction seems to occur more rapidly in distal intact organs than in the remnant liver after partial hepatectomy. HGF activity in the plasma after partial hepatectomy increased transiently within several hours and reached a peak after 24 hours [66]. DNA synthesis in the remnant liver increased to over 100-fold higher than that in the static phase (intact liver) at 24 hours after surgery (Fig. 3A). In addition to changes in HGF expression, *c-MET*/HGF receptors of plasma membranes prepared from the regenerating liver were down-regulated within several hours by internalization (endocytosis) after the binding of HGF. Importantly, this down-regulation of the receptor was specifically observed in the injured organ, but not in intact organs (Fig. 3B) [44].

In immunohistochemical analyses of liver regeneration, using incorporation of 5-bromo-2′-deoxyuridine (BrdU), cells undergoing DNA synthesis were distributed diffusely in the CCl_4-injured liver, while in the remnant liver after partial hepatectomy, cells undergoing DNA synthesis were distributed around the periportal area (zone 1), an area through which the arterio-portal blood inflows into liver lobules (Fig. 4).

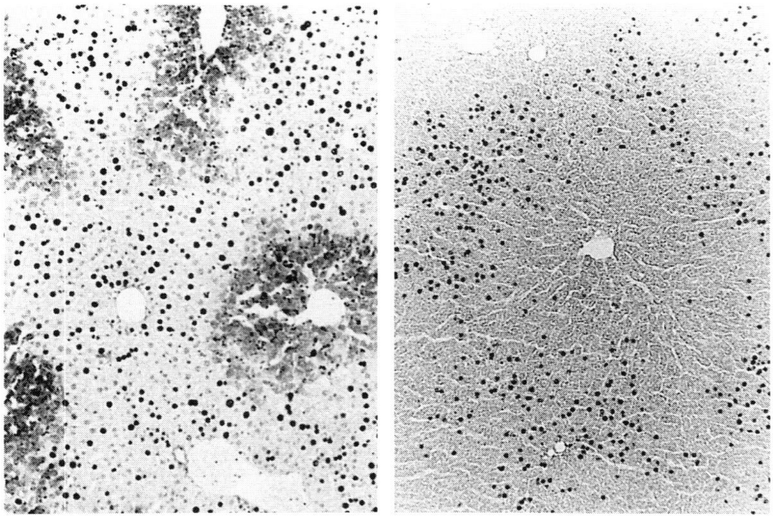

Fig. 4. Distribution of cells undergoing DNA synthesis in murine liver after CCl_4 administration or partial hepatectomy. In the case of CCl_4-induced hepatitis, the labeled cells undergoing DNA synthesis are distributed diffusely in the liver (left), whereas the labeled cells were predominantly located in zone 1 in the remnant liver after 30% partial hepatectomy (right).

These results suggest that there are two distinct mechanisms, paracrine and endocrine, involved in liver regeneration after liver injury (reviewed in [16]).

Regulation of HGF expression/induction

Based on the finding that the induction of HGF expression occurs in intact distal organs such as the lung and spleen in response to injuries, the presence of humoral factor which stimulates the expression of HGF mRNA in distal organs was considered. We detected such a humoral factor in the plasma of CCl_4-administered rats and named it "injurin" based on its biological function to mediate organ regeneration after injury [73]. During the purification of injurin, we found that several well-characterized factors have the potential to induce HGF expression. Cytokines such as interleukin-1 (IL-1) and tumor necrosis factor-α (TNF-α), and heparin are molecules possessing "injurin activity". IL-1 and TNF-α are strong inducers of HGF mRNA in human skin fibroblasts [74], while heparin is a strong enhancer of HGF protein, at the posttranscriptional level [75]. Recently, some prostanoids (prostaglandin E_1, I_2) were also shown to have potent "injurin activity" for the induction of

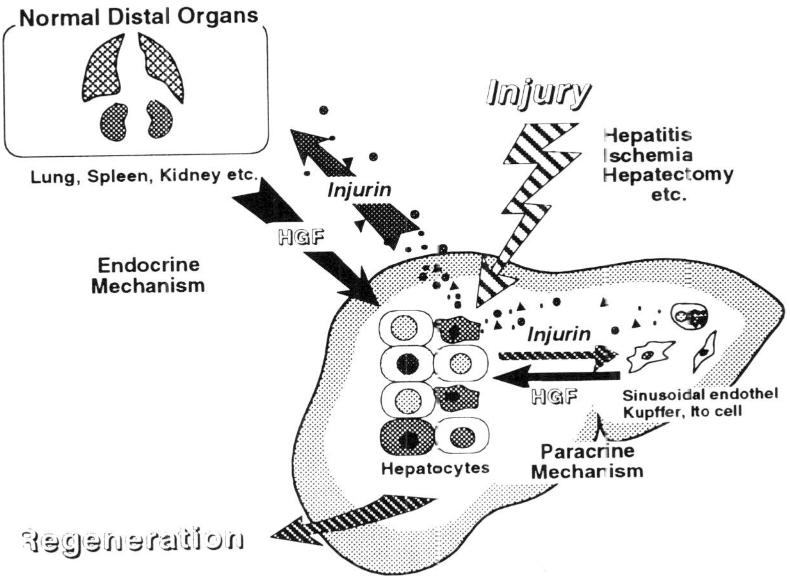

Fig. 5. Putative mechanisms of the initiation of liver regeneration by HGF/injurin.

HGF mRNA [76]. These factors may be rapidly and locally induced after organ injury, and induce HGF expression in impaired organs and also in distal intact organs. The putative mechanism for the initiation of liver regeneration by HGF is schematically described in Fig. 5.

Cells in various tissues and organs cease growth at later stages during the course of normal tissue repair. Regenerated tissues express differentiated functions, and there is a series of regenerative processes. Therefore, mechanisms related to the termination of regeneration of tissues and organs are as important as those for initiation of tissue regeneration. We found that transforming growth factor-β_1 (TGF-β_1) and glucocorticoids are potent negative regulators of HGF gene expression [77]. TGF-β_1 is also a potent growth suppressor for hepatocytes [78] and thus is considered to play an important role in the termination of liver regeneration.

In the case of chronic active hepatitis, tissue destruction and repair are chronically prolonged due to chronic inflammatory reactions and such a condition will lead to the onset of liver fibrosis. This pathophysiological condition does provide important insight into the mechanisms related to initiation and termination of liver regeneration. The expression of TGF-β_1 is remarkably and persistently up-regulated in a liver with a pathology [79,80]. Features leading to up-regulation of TGF-β_1 expression are unclear. Disorders (or imbalance) in the cytokine network (i.e. hyperexpression of inflammatory cytokines) may occur during prolonged inflammation due to

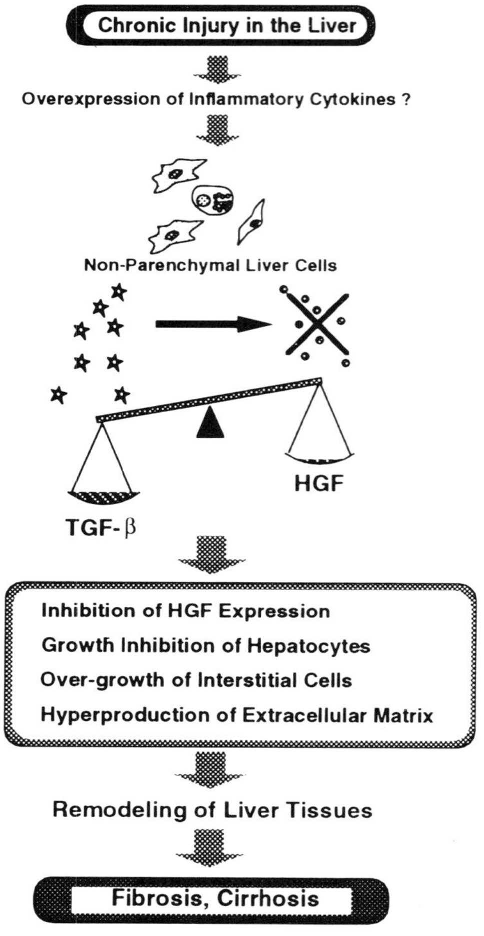

Fig. 6. A suggested mechanism of liver fibrosis and cirrhosis caused by the overexpression of TGF-β.

allergic reactions to viral antigen and to chemical reactions based on the toxicity of alcohol, and so on. Consequently, nonparenchymal liver cells such as Kupffer and Ito cells may be activated and the overproduction of TGF-β_1 may occur. Overexpression of TGF-β_1 suppresses the production of HGF, inhibits hepatocyte replication, and stimulates production of the extracellular matrix [77–80]. When such an overexpression of TGF-β_1 continues, impaired hepatocyte replication, enhanced deposition of extracellular matrix molecules, and overgrowth of nonparenchymal cells may occur, resulting in the onset of liver fibrosis (Fig. 6).

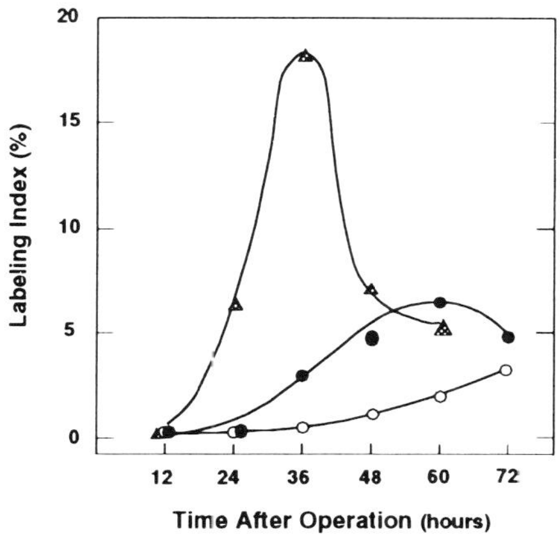

Fig. 7. Mitogenic effect of human recombinant HGF in vivo on liver regeneration after 30% partial hepatectomy in mice [81]. DNA synthesis in the remnant liver was determined by BrdU incorporation into hepatocytes. Administration of human recombinant HGF remarkably stimulated the DNA synthesis and facilitated the regeneration of remnant liver, in a dose-dependent manner. ○, control ; ●, mice given 1 μg HGF; △, mice given 5 μg HGF.

HGF as a potential therapeutic for liver diseases

In vivo organotrophic function of hr-HGF for liver regeneration

When human recombinant HGF (hr-HGF) was injected every 12 hours through the mouse tail vein after 30% partial hepatectomy, HGF elicited strong mitogenic effects in vivo (Fig. 7) [81]. In control mice injected with saline alone, DNA synthesis in the remnant liver increased from 36 to 72 hours after surgery. On the other hand, DNA synthesis reached the maximal level at 60 hours after operation, when injected with 1 μg/body (50 μg/kg) and the level was 3× higher than that of control mice. In the case of 5 μg/body of hr-HGF, DNA synthesis reached the maximal level at 36 hours after surgery and the maximal labeling index increased to 18%. These results indicate that DNA synthesis in the remnant liver was stimulated by HGF in a dose-dependent manner and liver regeneration was completed in a much shorter period than in the natural course. The possible clinical application of HGF to prevent hepatic failure after hepatectomy in patients with poor liver function is being considered.

Anti-inflammatory effects of HGF on biliary tract

Administration of α-naphthylisothiocyanate (ANIT) causes severe hepatobiliary cell necrosis 3 days later and enzymes from the liver, such as alanine aminotransferase (ALT), lactate dehydrogenase (LDH), alkaline phosphatase

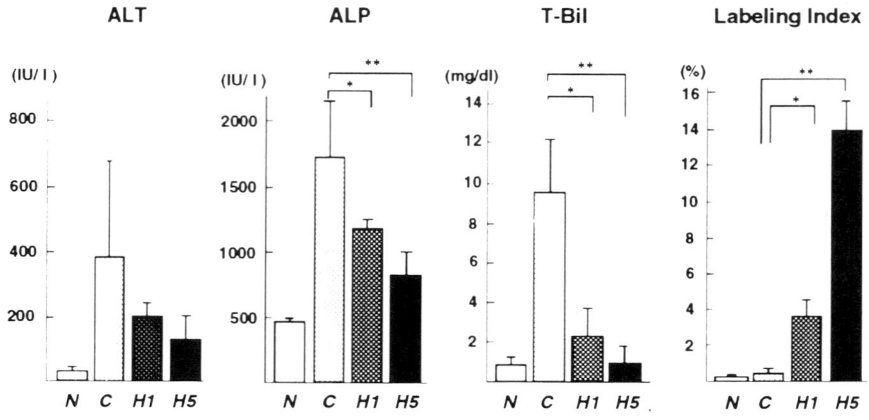

Fig. 8. Preventive effect of human recombinant HGF on the biliary tract injury caused by α-naphthylisothiocyanate (ANIT) in mice [81]. [ALT], alanine aminotransferase, [ALP], alkaline phosphatase, [T-Bil], serum total bilirubin, N, normal mice; C, control mice; H1, mice given 1 μg HGF; H5, mice given 5 μg HGF.

(ALP), leucine aminopeptidase (LAP), and total bilirubin (T-Bil), increase remarkably, as shown in Fig. 8. However, the concomitant administration of HGF strongly abrogated the degree of necrosis and the elevation in deviated enzymes [81]. Because HGF elicits mitogenic and morphogenic action not only for hepatocytes but also for biliary tract cells [64], HGF seems to stimulate the regeneration of hepato-biliary cells in an injured liver. Thus, HGF might directly prevent the cell damage caused by ANIT, because the pharmacological effects of HGF were apparent within 3 days.

Anticirrhotic action of hr-HGF

Liver cirrhosis can be induced in rats by the repeated intraperitoneal administration of dimethylnitrosamine (DMN). Liver fibrosis caused by DMN gradually progresses to the liver cirrhosis, resulting in severe hepatic failure. However, administration of 200 μg/kg hr-HGF into the DMN-administered rats stimulated tissue remodeling of the cirrhotic liver and prevented the progress of liver fibrosis/cirrhosis (unpublished data). These results suggest the possible clinical application of hr-HGF as a therapeutic for patients with liver cirrhosis.

HGF as an organotrophic factor

Compensatory hypertrophy of the kidney after unilateral nephrectomy is one phenomenon related to organ regeneration. We obtained evidence that HGF acts as a renotrophic factor for renal regeneration [20,21,82]. Unilateral nephrectomy in rats leads to a rapid induction of HGF mRNA in the remaining kidney, within several hours. HGF activity in the kidney reached a peak 12 hours after treatment, and DNA synthesis of renal tubular cells increased gradually and reached a peak 48 hours after surgery [21].

Concomitantly injected hr-HGF remarkably suppressed nephrotoxicity of aminoglycoside antibiotics (gentamicin), a potent anticancer drug (cisplatin) [82], and a potent immunosuppressant (cyclosporine) (unpublished data). These drugs elicit nephrotoxicity in some cases, because the effective concentration is close to the toxic dose, and toxicity sometimes has no therapeutic application in clinical cases. However, concomitant administration of hr-HGF prevented or reduced their side effects in in vivo experiments on animal models. Therefore, HGF may prove to be a safe and effective treatment for patients on these drugs. Likewise, HGF has an important role in the pulmonary regeneration. HGF mRNA rapidly increased to much higher levels than normal after the administration of HCl into the bronchoalveolar space, HGF activity and DNA synthesis in the lung then increased markedly [22].

Thus, HGF has a role in the regeneration of liver, kidney and lung. HGF is apparently an organotrophic factor which has important roles in organ regeneration.

Conclusion

HGF is the long-sought hepatotrophic factor for liver regeneration, and is now considered to be a pleiotropic factor which targets a wide variety of cells. HGF has crucial roles in organogenesis, morphogenesis, and regeneration of injured organs, because of its unique biological activities as mitogen, motogen, and morphogen. HGF is expected to contribute not only to elucidation of the pathogenesis of disease but may also prove to be a diagnostic and a factor which can be added to the armamentarium of therapeutic agents.

Acknowledgements

We thank M. Ohara for assistance in preparing the manuscript and all our colleagues for assistance in carrying out HGF-related investigations, in particular the physiological analysis of organ regeneration. Our studies have been supported by a research grant for Science and Cancer from the Ministry of Education, Science, and Culture of Japan and research grants from the Uehara Foundation, Ysasuda Memorial Foundation, and Mochida Memorial Foundation.

References

1. Nakamura T, Nawa K, Ichihara A. Biohem Biophys Res Commun 1984;122:1450–1459.
2. Russell WE, McGowan JA, Bucher NLR. J Cell Physiol 1984;119:183–192.
3. Michalopoulos G, Houck KA, Dolan ML et al. Cancer Res 1984;44:4414–4419.
4. Matsumoto K, Nakamura T. Crit Rev Oncogenesis 1992;3:27–54.
5. Nakamura T, Teramoto H, Ichihara A. Proc Natl Acad Sci USA 1986;83:6489–6493.
6. Nakamura T, Nawa K, Ichihara A et al. FEBS Lett 1987;224:311–316.
7. Nakamura T, Nishizawa T, Hagiya M et al. Nature 1989;342:440–443.
8. Seki T, Ihara I, Sugiura A et al. Biochem Biophys Res Commun 1990;172:321–327.
9. Tashiro K, Hagiya M, Nishizawa T et al. Proc Natl Acad Sci USA 1990;87:3200–3204.
10. Miyazawa K, Tsubouchi H, Naka D et al. Biochem Biophys Res Commun 1989;163:967–973.
11. Ghoda E, Tsubouchi H, Nakayama H et al. J Clin Invest 1988;81:414–419.
12. Zarnegar R, Michalopoulos GK. Cancer Res 1989;49:3314–3320.
13. Rubin JS, Chan AML, Bottaro DP et al. Proc Natl Acad Sci USA 1991;88:415–419.
14. Montesano R, Matsumoto K, Nakamura T et al. Cell 1991;67:901–908.
15. Gherardi E, Stoker M. Cancer Cell 1991;3:227–232.
16. Weidner KM, Behrens J, Vandekerckhove J et al. J Cell Biol 1990;111:2097–2108.
17. Matsumoto K, Nakamura T. In: Goldberg ID, Rosen EM (eds) Hepatocyte Growth Factor-Scatter Factor (HGF-SF) and the C-MET Receptor. Basel: Birkhäuser Verlag, 1993;225–249.
18. Matsumoto K, Nakamura T. Gann Monograph 1994;42:91–112.
19. Kinoshita T, Tashiro K, Nakamura T. Biochem Biophys Res Commun 1989;165:1229–1234.
20. Igawa T, Matsumoto K, Kanda S et al. Am J Physiol 1993;265:F61–F69.
21. Nagaike M, Hirao S, Tajima H et al. J Biol Chem 1991;266:22781–22784.
22. Yanagita K, Matsumoto K, Sekiguchi K et al. J Biol Chem 1993;268:21212–21217.
23. Di Renzo MF, Narsimhan RP, Olivero M et al. Oncogene 1991;6:1997–2003.
24. Tajima H, Matsumoto K, Nakamura T. FEBS Lett 1991;291:229–232.
25. Shima N, Nagao M, Ogaki F et al. Biochem Biophys Res Commun 1991:180;1151–1158.
26. Higashio K, Shima N, Goto M et al. Biochem Biophys Res Commun 1991;170:397–404.
27. Shiota G, Rhoads DB, Wang TC et al. Proc Natl Acad Sci USA 1992;89:373–377.
28. Defrances MC, Wolf HK, Michalopoulos GK et al. Development 1992;116:387–395.
29. Santos OF, Barros EJG, Yang XM et al. Develop Biol 1994;163:525–529.
30. Stern CD, Ireland GW, Herrick SE et al. Development 1990;110:1271–1284.
31. Tsubouchi H, Niitani Y, Hirono S et al. Hepatology 1991;13:1–5.
32. Chang H, Nagao T, Ichikawa N et al. Nephron 1994;67:497–498.
33. Kmiecik TE, Keller JR, Rosen E et al. Blood 1992;80:2454–2457.
34. Mizuno K, Higuchi O, Ihle JN et al. Biochem Biophys Res Commun 1993;194:178–186.
35. Takebayashi T, Iwamoto M, Jikko A et al. Hepatocyte growth factor/scatter factor has mitogenic, motogenic, and morphogenic activity on chondrocytes. J Cell Biol (in press).
36. Cooper CS, Park M, Blair DG et al. Nature 1984:311;29–33.
37. Bottaro DP, Rubin JS, Faletto DL et al. Science 1991;251:802–804.
38. Naldini L, Vigna E, Narsimham RP et al. Oncogene 1991;6:501–504.
39. Higuchi O, Mizuno K, Van de Woude GF et al. FEBS Lett 1992;301:282–286.
40. Park M, Dean M, Kaul K et al. Proc Natl Acad Sci USA 1987;84:6379–6383.
41. Naldini L, Weidner KM, Vigna E et al. EMBO J 1991;10:2867–2878.
42. Ponzetto C, Bardelli A, Zhen Z et al. Cell 1994;77:261–271.
43. Higuchi O, Nakamura T. Biochem Biophys Res Commun 1991;176:599–607.
44. Tajima H, Higuchi O, Mizuno K et al. J Biochem 1992;111:401–406.
45. Tajima H, Matsumoto K, Nakamura T. Exp Cell Res 1992;202:423-431.
46. Mizuno K, Inoue H, Hagiya M et al. J Biol Chem 1994;269:1131–1136.

47. Lyon M, Deakin JA, Mizuno K et al. J Biol Chem 1994;269:11216–11223.
48. Masumoto A, Yamamoto N. Biochem Biophys Res Commun 1991;174:90–95.
49. Liu K, Kato Y, Narukawa M et al. Am J Physiol 1992;263:G642–G649.
50. Lokker NA, Mark MR, Luis EA et al. EMBO J 1992;11:2503–2510.
51. Matsumoto K, Takehara T, Inoue H et al. Biochem Biophys Res Commun 1991;181:691–699.
52. Fukuyama R, Ichijyo Y, Minoshima S et al. Genomics 1991;11:410–415.
53. Seki T, Hagiya M, Shimonishi M et al. Gene 1991;102:213–219.
54. Mizuno K, Tanoue Y, Okano I et al. Biochem Biophys Res Commun 1994;198:1161–1169.
55. Shimomura T, Ochiai M, Kondo J et al. Cytotechnology 1992,8:219–229.
56. Miyazawa K, Shimomura T, Kitamura A et al. J Biol Chem 1993;268:10024–10028.
57. Matsumoto K, Hashimoto K, Yoshikawa K et al. Exp Cell Res 1991;196:114–120.
58. Igawa T, Kanda S, Kanetake H et al. Biochem Biophys Res Commun 1991;174:831–838.
59. Mason RJ, Leslie CC, McCormick-Shannon K et al. Am J Respir Cell Mol Biol 1994;11:561–567.
60. Morimoto A, Okamura K, Hamanaka R et al. Biochem Biophys Res Commun 1991;179:1042–1049.
61. Bussolino F, DiRenzo MF, Ziche M et al. J Cell Biol 1992;119:629–641.
62. Furlong RA, Takehara T, Taylor WG et al. J Cell Sci 1991;100:173–177.
63. Weidner KM, Arakaki N, Hartmann G et al. Proc Natl Acad Sci USA 1991;88:7001–7005.
64. Johnson M, Koukoulis G, Matsumoto K et al. Hepatology 1993;17:1052–1061.
65. Hamanoue M, Kawaida K, Takao S et al. Hepatology 1992;16:1485–1492.
66. Kinoshita T, Hirao S, Matsumoto K et al. Biochem Biophys Res Commun 1991;177:330–335.
67. Lindroos PM, Zarnegar R, Michalopoulos GK. Hepatology 1991;13:734–750.
68. Noji S, Tashiro K, Koyoma E et al. Biochem Biophys Res Commun 1990;173:42–47.
69. Schirmacher P, Geerts A, Piertrangelo A et al. Hepatology 1992;15:5–11.
70. Ramadori G, Neubauer K, Odenthal M et al. Biochem Biophys Res Commun 1992;183:739–742.
71. Yanagita K, Nagaike M, Ishibashi H et al. Biochem Biophys Res Commun 1992;182:802–809.
72. Kono S, Nagaike M, Matsumoto K et al. Biochem Biophys Res Commun 1992;186:991–998.
73. Matsumoto K, Tajima H, Hamanoue M et al. Proc Natl Acad Sci USA 1992;89:3800–3804.
74. Matsumoto K, Okazaki H, Nakamura T. Biochem Biophys Res Commun 1992;188:235–243.
75. Matsumoto K, Tajima H, Okazaki H et al. J Biochem 1993;114:820–826.
76. Matsumoto K, Okazaki H, Nakamura T. J Biochem (in press).
77. Matsumoto K, Tajima H, Okazaki H et al. J Biol Chem 1992;267:24917–24920.
78. Nakamura T, Tomita Y, Hirai R et al. Biochem Biophys Res Commun 1985;133:1042–1050.
79. Czaja MJ, Weiner FR, Flanders KC et al. J Cell Biol 1989;108:2477–2482.
80. Nakatsukasa H, Nagy P, Evarts RP et al. J Clin Invest 1990;85:1833–1843.
81. Ishiki Y, Ohnishi H, Muto Y et al. Hepatology 1992;16:1227–1235.
82. Kawaida K, Matsumoto K, Shimazu H et al. Proc Natl Acad Sci USA 1994;91:4357–4361.

Progress in Hepatology Vol. 1.
Cellular and Molecular Biology.
M. Yamanaka, K. Okabe and G. Toda, editors.

Acute liver failure. Possible mechanisms of massive hepatic necrosis and impaired liver regeneration

Kenji Fujiwara[1], Satoshi Mochida[1], Tomoaki Tomiya[2], Keiichi Hirata[2], Sumiko Nagoshi[2], Akihiko Ohno[2], Masahiro Arai[2] and Itsuro Ogata[2]

[1]*Third Department of Internal Medicine, Saitama Medical School, Saitama 350-04; and* [2]*First Department of Internal Medicine, University of Tokyo, Tokyo 113, Japan*

Abstract. The mechanisms of massive hepatic necrosis and impaired liver regeneration in acute liver failure were investigated. Massive hepatic necrosis occurred as a result of fibrin deposition in the hepatic sinusoids through regulatory imbalance in coagulation between thrombomodulin expressed on the surface of sinusoidal endothelial cells and tissue factor generated by hepatic macrophages in rats. The reduction in thrombomodulin was produced by the endothelial cell damage due to fat-storing cell injury or activation of hepatic macrophages. There were two types of endothelial cell damage by activated hepatic macrophages: direct destruction by cytotoxic mediators and indirect destruction by fibrin deposition resulting from excessive tissue factor generation. Hepatocyte growth factor and epidermal growth factor produced liver growth in normal rats as well as partially hepatectomized rats. In liver plasma membrane, there was stimulatory activity as well as inhibitory activity on DNA synthesis induced by mitogens in cultured rat hepatocytes, suggesting that liver growth is regulated by the membrane together with mitogens. Serum-transforming growth factor α levels were increased in association with the extent of liver growth in patients after partial hepatectomy, and changed reflecting liver growth in rats. The levels were positively correlated with the extent of liver injury in patients with acute hepatitis, but this relationship was reversed in patients with acute liver failure. In nonsurvivors of those patients, the levels were gradually decreased until death, suggesting that there is impaired liver regeneration in fatal acute liver failure. In liver plasma membrane of carbon tetrachloride intoxicated rats, the stimulatory activity on DNA synthesis by cultured rat hepatocytes was lost even when the inhibitory activity was still present.

Key words: endothelial cell, epidermal growth factor, hepatic macrophage, hepatocyte growth factor, intravascular coagulation, liver regeneration, liver transplantation, plasma membrane, putrescine, thrombomodulin, tissue factor, transforming growth factor α.

Acute liver failure often takes a fatal course with encephalopathy and multiple organ failure [1]. Although the cause varies, massive or submassive hepatic necrosis is common, and sufficient liver regeneration is required for survival [2]. Thus, when liver dysfunction due to massive hepatic necrosis is

Address for correspondence: Kenji Fujiwara, M.D., Ph.D., Third Department of Internal Medicine, Saitama Medical School, Moroyama-machi, Iruma-gun, Saitama 350-04, Japan. Phone: 81-492-76-1198, Fax: 81-492-94-8404

severe enough to produce fatal metabolic disorders or liver regeneration is impaired, survival would fail.

To improve the survival rate of patients with acute liver failure, new modalities for treatment based on the mechanisms of massive hepatic necrosis and impaired liver regeneration are necessary. The present paper reports on experimental and clinical results regarding such matters in acute liver failure.

Massive hepatic necrosis

Regulatory mechanisms of coagulation in the hepatic sinusoids

Endothelial cells are considered to inhibit coagulation, because they generate a variety of antithrombogenic factors such as thrombomodulin, heparin-like substance, tissue factor pathway inhibitor, prostaglandin I_2 and tissue plasminogen activator [3]. Thrombomodulin is the most important of them, as it not only blocks thrombin function, but also as its complex with thrombin activates protein C to inactivate coagulation factors V and VIII [3]. On the other hand, macrophages are known to produce tissue factor [4–6] which acts as a trigger for coagulation [7], thus suggesting that coagulation in the hepatic sinusoids may be regulated by tissue factor released from hepatic macrophages and antithrombogenic factors expressed on the surface of sinusoidal endothelial cells, particularly thrombomodulin (Fig. 1).

When cryostat sections of frozen normal rat liver were stained by the avidin-biotin-peroxidase complex method using polyclonal antibody against human thrombomodulin as a primary antibody [8], thrombomodulin was expressed along endothelial cells slightly in the hepatic sinusoids and markedly in large vessels. The extent of this expression in the hepatic sinusoids was much less compared to that in alveolar capillaries of the lung [9,10]. Similar results were also seen when Northern blotting for thrombomo-

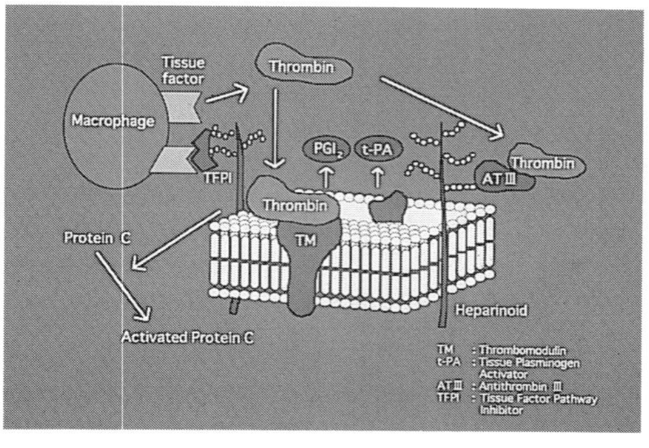

Fig. 1. Regulatory mechanisms of coagulation in the hepatic sinusoids.

dulin mRNA expression was studied with both organ tissues [11], suggesting that fibrin deposition can occur more easily in the hepatic sinusoids than in the capillaries of other organs.

Kupffer cells and pulmonary macrophages were isolated from normal rats, and cultured in the presence or absence of endotoxin. Then tissue factor activity was determined in the cells by the method of Hische et al. [12]. The activity in the presence of endotoxin was significantly higher than that in the absence of endotoxin in both cells, but its extent was much less in Kupffer cells than in pulmonary macrophages [10]. These results may explain the fact that coagulopathy seldom develops on the surface of sinusoidal endothelial cells in normal liver although they express less thrombomodulin and Kupffer cells are always exposed to stimulating substances derived from the gut.

Sinusoidal fibrin deposition as a cause of massive hepatic necrosis

Liver damage was induced in rats by injection of carbon tetrachloride (CCl_4) or dimethylnitrosamine (DMN). Although prothrombin time was similarly prolonged in both groups, plasma levels of soluble fibrin monomer complex were significantly higher in the DMN group than in the CCl_4 group [13]. Electron microscopic examination revealed that fibrin deposition was present only in the necrotic areas in the CCl_4 group, but observed in the hepatic sinusoids as well as in the necrotic areas in the DMN group [13]. Infusion with antithrombin III (AT III) concentrated attenuated derangements of serum total bilirubin and ALT levels in a dose-related manner only in the DNM group [13]. Severe coagulopathy occurring in the liver may be associated with fibrin deposition in the hepatic sinusoids which produced massive hepatic necrosis.

Electron microscopic examination serially performed after intoxication disclosed that sinusoidal fibrin deposition in the DMN group occurred following endothelial cell destruction and the initial abnormal finding was apoptosis of fat-storing cells which reinforce the sinusoidal wall. In contrast, endothelial cells remained intact in the CCl_4 group [14]. The development of endothelial cell destruction in the DMN group was also supported by alterations in plasma levels of fibrinogen and coagulation factor VIII:C which is exclusively produced by endothelial cells [14], suggesting that endothelial cell damage is essential to the development of fibrin deposition in the hepatic sinusoids.

Mechanisms of sinusoidal fibrin deposition induced by activated hepatic macrophages

It is well known that massive hepatic necrosis is induced by endotoxin administration in rodents given heat-killed *Corynebacterium parvum* [15]. Similar necrosis was provoked by endotoxin administration after partial hepatectomy in rats [16,17]. According to the method of liver perfusion with nitro blue tetrazolium and phorbol myristate acetate which can determine in situ the ability of hepatic macrophages to produce superoxide anions [18–20], formazan deposition reflecting superoxide anion production was markedly seen in hepatic macrophages throughout the liver following partial hepatectomy as well as *C. parvum* administration in rats [16,19,21]. The extent of formazan deposition was reduced by pretreatment with gum arabic, a polysaccharide of high molecular weight which can block macrophage function [16,22].

When massive hepatic necrosis occurred after endotoxin administration, there was fibrin deposition and endothelial cell destruction in the hepatic sinusoids in both models [16,23]. Infusion with AT III concentrate or pretreatment with gum arabic markedly attenuated both liver injuries [16,23]. However, when those rats were treated with superoxide dismutase or anti-TNFα antibody, the attenuation was seen only in the *C. parvum* model [11,16,23]. Eradication of circulating neutrophils by polyclonal antibody did not cause any effect in both models [11]. Thus, activated hepatic macrophages are considered to contribute to the development of both liver injuries, but macrophage-derived mediators reponsible for the injury seem to differ between both models.

Purine nucleoside phosphorylase (PNP) is present in hepatocytes as well as in sinusoidal endothelial cells, but ALT is found exclusively in hepatocytes [24,25]. In *C. parvum*-treated rats and partially hepatectomized rats, the activities of TNF, PNP and ALT were serially measured in serum following endotoxin administration, and compared with those activities in the perfusate during closed liver perfusion with DMEM containing fetal calf serum and endotoxin. Serum activities of PNP and ALT were successively increased following a transient increase in TNF activity in *C. parvum*-treated rats [24]. PNP activity was also increased in the perfusate, but ALT activity remained unchanged [24]. This increase of PNP activity was significantly attenuated by pretreatment of rats with gadolinium chloride which suppresses hepatic macrophage function [24]. In contrast, PNP and ALT activities were similarly increased in serum, but not in the perfusate in partially hepatectomized rats [11]. In this model, serum TNF concentration was 10^4 times lower than that in the *C. parvum* model [11]. These results may suggest that activated macrophages in the *C. parvum* model directly destroyed endothelial cells by releasing cytotoxic mediators, but such a mechanism did not operate in the partial hepatectomy model. Since blood coagulation never occurs in the perfused liver, sinusoidal endothelial cell damage in vivo in the partial hepatectomy model seems to be the result of fibrin deposition in the hepatic sinusoids.

Tissue factor activity was measured in hepatic macrophages isolated from rats given *C. parvum* or after partial hepatectomy and cultured in the presence or absence of endotoxin. The activity was much higher after partial hepatectomy than after *C. parvum* administration in the absence as well as in the presence of endotoxin [11], suggesting that coagulopathy can be triggered by excitation of hepatic macrophages more easily after partial hepatectomy than after *C. parvum* administration. When recombinant thrombomodulin was dosed to rats after partial hepatectomy, the deranged serum ALT activity was significantly attenuated compared to the controls [11]. Similar results were also obtained when recombinant tissue factor pathway inhibitor was used. Thus, it is concluded that endothelial cells are destroyed by cytotoxic mediators including TNFα released from hepatic macrophages after excitation with endotoxin in *C. parvum*-treated rats. In partially hepatectomized rats, the regulation of coagulation in the hepatic sinusoids is deranged by increased tissue factor activity to form fibrin deposition leading to endothelial cell destruction.

When the immunohistochemical expression of ICAM-1 and LFA-1 in the liver was studied in both models, their expression was significantly increased compared to normal liver. The cells expressing ICAM-1 and LFA-1 were electron-microscopically identified as endothelial cells and macrophages, respectively [11]. Therapy with monoclonal antibodies against rat ICAM-1 and LFA-1α significantly attenuated the extent of liver injury in the *C. parvum* model compared to the control, but the effect was reversed in the partial hepatectomy model [11]. It seems that the adhesion of hepatic macrophages to sinusoidal endothelial cells increases cytotoxic mediators on the surface of the endothelial cells in the *C. parvum* model, whereas antithrombogenic factors expressed on the surface of the endothelial cells effectively reduce coagulopathy induced by excessive tissue factor on the surface of hepatic macrophages in the partial hepatectomy model.

These results may indicate that there are two types of endothelial cell damage related to activated macrophages in the hepatic sinusoids. One is that superoxide anions and TNFα released from the macrophages directly destroy endothelial cells, resulting in loss of thrombomodulin activity, and the other is that the macrophages produce insufficient amounts of both cytotoxic mediators, but abundant tissue factor leads to an increase in thrombin generation. The role of both cell contact via ICAM-1 and LFA-1 in the development of this coagulopathy is reversed in both types of endothelial cell damage (Fig. 2).

Mechanisms of injury in the liver transplanted following cold preservation

When rat liver was preserved at 1°C in University of Wisconsin (UW) solution, endothelial cell disruption developed after 12 h and endothelial cell detachment into the lumen after 18 h. This detachment was accompanied by fat-storing cell degeneration. Both cell abnormalities were parallel to each other in degree [26], suggesting that fat-storing cell damage may cause endothelial cell detachment.

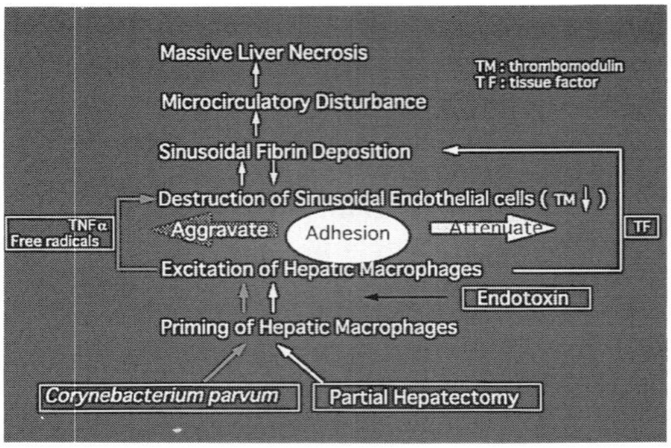

Fig. 2. Mechanisms of sinusoidal fibrin deposition induced by activated hepatic macrophages.

Immunohistochemical study revealed that thrombomodulin expression was much less in the sinusoidal walls in preserved liver compared with normal liver. This decreased expression in the preserved liver remained even after transplantation [10].

The stimulatory state of hepatic macrophages in the liver after cold preservation was determined according to the method of liver perfusion with nitro blue tetrazolium was remarkably activated [25]. On the other hand, tissue factor activity in hepatic macrophages isolated 1 h after transplantation of the liver was significantly increased irrespective of the duration of preservation compared to normal liver [10]. When these macrophages were cultured for 5 h in the presence of endotoxin, the activity was further elevated, but its extent was significantly greater in the transplanted liver than in normal liver [10].

When the liver transplanted following cold preservation in UW solution for 24 h was electron-microscopically observed 5 h after surgery, there was fibrin deposition in the hepatic sinusoids which showed strands with a longitudinal periodicity of 23 nm under greater magnification [27]. Infusion with AT III concentrate immediately and 12 h after transplantation attenuated deranged levels of serum ALT and plasma AT III 24 h after transplantation [27].

From these results, it is clear that the hypercoagulative state in the hepatic sinusoids is present after transplantation of the preserved liver. The derangement of coagulation equilibrium regulated by tissue factor derived from activated macrophages and thrombomodulin expressed on the surface of endothelial cells may cause such coagulopathy as is found in massive hepatic necrosis produced by endotoxin following *C. parvum* administration or partial hepatectomy. Fat-storing cell damage would also contribute to the aggravation of this state through reduction in the number of endothelial cells.

Impaired liver regeneration

Role of mitogens in the regulation of liver growth

When 100 μg/kg body weight of hepatocyte growth factor (HGF) was intravenously injected in normal rats, serum HGF concentrations at 30 min and 2 h later were 22 and 3 ng/ml, respectively [28], suggesting that HGF doses at 2-h intervals can maintain serum HGF concentrations enough to stimulate hepatocyte proliferation in vitro.

HGF at this dose was similarly injected at 2-h intervals for 10 h to normal rats or partially hepatectomized rats starting immediately after operation, and hepatic DNA content was measured 48 h after the start of HGF administration. Hepatic DNA content was increased by HGF administration in normal rats as well as in partially hepatectomized rats [28].

It is well known that polyamines are involved in cell growth, particularly that putrescine is essential for liver regeneration at its early stage after partial hepatectomy [29]. Putrescine is synthesized from ornithine by action of ornithine decarboxylase (ODC) or via a compensatory route from spermidine by action of spermidine N1-acetyltransferase (SAT) [30]. Hepatic putrescine content and ODC and SAT activities were measured in those rats 6 h after the start of HGF administration. HGF administration significantly increased the putrescine content and both enzyme activities in normal rats almost to the levels after partial hepatectomy [28]. Those levels in partially hepatectomized rats were further enhanced by HGF administration [28]. This result may indicate that exogenous HGF produced polyamine metabolism similar to regenerating liver in normal liver.

When 5-bromo-2′-deoxyuridine labeling index and mitotic index of hepatocytes and hepatic DNA content were determined at different time points until 48 h in normal rats given HGF, both indices were significantly increased by HGF administration at 26 h, followed by a significant increase in hepatic DNA content. The labeled hepatocytes in HGF-treated rats were present in the periportal and midzonal areas of lobules [28].

From these results, it is concluded that exogenous HGF acts as a trigger as well as a promoter of liver growth. Similar results in normal liver were also seen when epidermal growth factor (EGF) was used instead of HGF [31].

According to cell contact inhibition theory, hepatocyte proliferation should be inhibited by cell-surface modulators of hepatocytes in normal liver [32–34]. Thus, the present results that such doses of HGF or EGF produced overgrowth of normal liver may suggest that the potency of HGF or EGF in stimulating hepatocyte proliferation overcame the strength of such cell-surface modulators. To verify this hypothesis, HGF at varying concentrations was added to the culture medium of rat hepatocytes in the presence or absence of plasma membrane purified from the liver, and DNA synthesis by the cells was measured. The DNA synthesis was increased by addition of HGF in a dose-related manner, but this increase was depressed by addition of the plasma membrane. However, the DNA synthesis was increased to some extent at high concentrations of HGF even in the presence of the plasma membrane [28].

Regulation of liver regeneration by liver plasma membrane

Protein kinase C is known to play a role in rendering resting cells into a competent state to proliferate. EGF and insulin were added to the medium of rat hepatocytes in primary culture 6 h after plating hepatocytes, and DNA synthesis by the cells was measured at 30 h. The DNA synthesis was much smaller than the DNA synthesis induced by EGF and insulin added at 24 h and measured at 50 h, but significantly increased by pretreatment of the cells with vasopressin or TPA [34]. This increase was inhibited by liver plasma membrane added at 2 h of plating. The DNA synthesis was also decreased by addition of H-7, an inhibitor of protein kinases A, C and G, and also by HA-1004, an inhibitor of protein kinases A and G. The decrease by H-7 was significantly greater than that by H-1004 [34]. From these results, it is concluded that DNA synthesis induction by EGF and insulin may require a priming period related to protein kinase C activation in cultured rat hepatocytes, and liver plasma membrane inhibits this process.

In an extension of these experiments, we have found unexpectedly that the plasma membrane promotes DNA synthesis by cultured rat hepatocytes as well under certain experimental conditions. EGF and insulin were added to the culture medium 24 h after plating, and DNA synthesis was assayed at 50 h. When the plasma membrane was added before 24 h, the DNA synthesis was significantly decreased, compared to controls, but increased by its addition at 30 or 38 h. DNA synthesis at 50 h was negligible in the absence of EGF and insulin even when the plasma membrane was added at 38 h. When the plasma membrane was added immediately after EGF and insulin were removed from the culture medium at 38 h by washing, the increase in DNA synthesis became much smaller, but was restored by further addition of EGF and insulin immediately following the washing [35].

These results indicate that the plasma membrane contains not only an inhibitory factor but also a stimulatory factor for DNA synthesis by rat hepatocytes in primary culture, and this stimulatory factor is a comitogen for hepatocyte proliferation. Such inhibitory and stimulatory effects of the plasma membrane were also seen when HGF was used instead of EGF.

The stimulatory activity of the plasma membrane was found in the supernatant from the plasma membrane after collagenase digestion, and detectable in its fraction with molecular weight less than 25 kD. The factor seems to be protein in character because the activity was lost by heating or acid treatment [35].

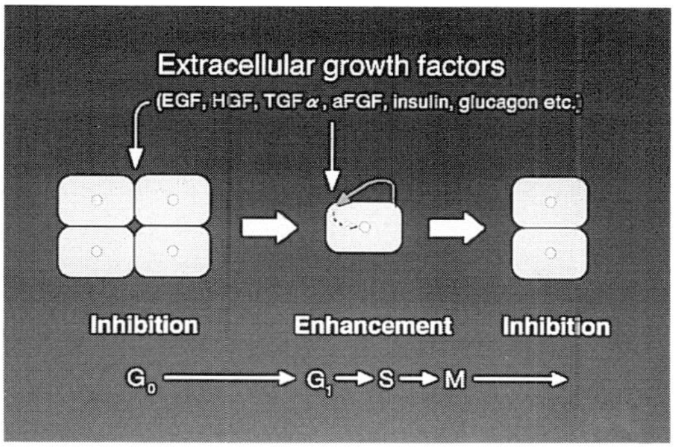

Fig. 3. Mechanisms of liver regeneration.

Proposed mechanisms of liver regeneration

Based on these experimental results, a tentative hypothesis regarding the regulatory mechanisms of liver regeneration is proposed as follows. The liver is always exposed to a variety of factors with potential to promote hepatocyte proliferation. The potentialities of such factors vary depending on the environment. In normal liver the inhibitory activity of plasma membrane can overcome these potentialities. When the inhibitory activity of adjacent hepatocyte plasma membrane is decreased as a result of loss of contact with each other by partial resection or necrosis, such factors will potentially become enough to stimulate proliferation. The increasing amount of mitogens such as HGF and TGFα would additionally promote this process. The stimulatory factor of plasma membrane will also participate in such promotion as a comitogen (Fig. 3).

Significance of increased serum levels of HGF and TGFα

HGF

Serum HGF levels were measured in patients with hepatic failure of fulminant and chronic types. The levels were abnormally increased in all patients with fulminant hepatic failure and in most patients with chronic hepatic failure. The levels in the fulminant failure group were significantly higher than those in the chronic hepatic failure group, even when serum HGF levels were compared by matching the severity of hepatic failure in both groups with prothrombin time and coma grade [36]. In patients with chronic liver disease, serum HGF levels were negatively correlated with prothrombin time (% of normal) and serum levels of albumin and cholinesterase, and positively correlated with serum levels of total bilirubin, total bile acid and AST. The correlation with serum AST levels was more prominent in patients whose prothrombin time was within normal range. In these patients, serum HGF levels were also positively correlated with serum ALT [36].

When serum HGF levels were measured in patients with chronic renal failure who had no liver disease, the levels were abnormally increased in 44% of the patients, and significantly elevated immediately after hemodialysis using heparin in all patients [36].

Serum HGF levels were measured in 14 hepatectomized and 10 nonhepatectomized surgical patients. In the hepatectomized group, seven patients had hepatocellular carcinoma with liver cirrhosis and seven had metastatic liver tumor with no chronic liver disease. Serum HGF levels were elevated after surgery and reached a maximum within seven days in all patients of the hepatectomized group irrespective of the presence of liver cirrhosis. The levels decreased gradually thereafter and returned to preoperative values until 28 days after surgery. A similar increase in serum HGF levels after surgery was also seen in the nonhepatectomized group, but recovery to preoperative levels occurred earlier [37]. When the maximal HGF levels after surgery were analyzed by multiple regression model, postoperative maximal serum HGF levels were significantly and independently related to the presence of liver cirrhosis, postoperative maximal serum total bilirubin and ALT levels, and peripheral white blood cell counts in the hepatectomized group. However, there was no relationship between such HGF levels and percent resected liver volume or increment of the remaining liver volume 28 days after partial hepatectomy. In the nonhepatectomized group, postoperative maximal serum HGF levels had significant and independent relationships with postoperative peripheral white blood cell counts and serum C-reactive protein levels [37].

It is concluded that serum HGF levels were increased in association with hepatocellular dysfunction and necrosis and systemic inflammation. Renal failure and extracorporeal circulation using heparin as an anticoagulant may also increase serum HGF levels. It is unlikely that the increase was related to liver regeneration.

TGFα

We have developed a simple and reliable sandwich ELISA to measure serum TGFα levels with monoclonal IgM and polyclonal IgG antihuman TGFα antibodies and a system to amplify the activity-conjugated enzymes which detects serum TGFα levels as low as 5 pg/ml without condensation or deproteinization of samples [38].

When serum TGFα levels were measured with this method in 13 patients who underwent partial hepatectomy for hepatocellular carcinoma with liver cirrhosis, the levels before surgery were significantly higher in patients who underwent partial hepatectomy than in healthy adults. Although the levels transiently decreased within 7 days after surgery in 54% of patients, the maximal levels in each case within 28 days were higher than the levels before surgery. The maximal levels within 28 days of surgery showed no significant relationship to age, sex, type of tumor or presence of cirrhosis [38]. Those maximal levels were correlated significantly with percent resected liver volume and percent increased volume of the remaining liver calculated on CT imagings 28 days after surgery. In contrast, the levels showed no increase after laparotomy for nonhepatic surgery [38]. Serum TGFα levels may vary depending on the regenerative stimulus and reflect the degree to which liver regeneration will occur in patients after partial hepatectomy.

This possibility was studied with animal experiments. Three models of liver growth were induced in rats, and TGFα levels were determined in the liver and serum. When rats underwent two-thirds resection of the liver, TGFα levels in the liver were gradually increased until 24 h after operation, and then gradually decreased to the preoperative levels at 96 h Serum TGFα levels changed together with those changes in the liver. Serum TGFα levels are likely to reflect TGFα production by regenerating liver [39]. The second model was made by administration of CCl_4. Serum TGFα levels were increased following the elevation of serum ALT levels, with the similar changes in TGFα levels and mitotic index in the liver [39]. When rats were given phenobarbital in drinking water, TGFα levels in the liver and serum gradually increased from 3 days. In this model, liver weight and the number of mitotic hepatocytes also increased from 3 days [39].

From these results, it is concluded that serum TGFα is originated from TGFα in the liver which increases in association with liver growth.

Impaired liver regeneration in acute liver failure

Serum TGFα levels were measured in serial time points in 19 patients with acute hepatitis and 20 patients with fulminant hepatic failure. In most of the acute hepatitis group, serum TGFα levels were abnormally increased, but half in the fulminant hepatic failure group showed the levels within normal range [40].

In those patients with fulminant hepatic failure, there was no correlation between serum TGFα levels and HGF levels. However, all patients who had abnormally increased serum TGFα levels showed serum HGF levels below 5 ng/ml [40].

Serum TGFα levels were serially measured in nonsurvivors with fulminant hepatic failure until death. In those patients, even when serum TGFα levels were high during the course, the levels were gradually decreased [40].

In patients with acute hepatitis, serum TGFα levels were positively correlated with serum ALT and total bilirubin levels. In contrast, this relationship with serum total bilirubin levels was reversed in patients with fulminant hepatic failure [40].

From those results, it is strongly suggested that liver regeneration is insufficient in patients with fulminant hepatic failure, particularly when patients are mortally ill.

When plasma membrane was obtained from rat liver after CCl_4 intoxication, its stimulatory activity was decreased with the development of liver damage. However, the inhibitory activity was maintained when 30% of the stimulatory activity was lost, suggesting that EGF and HGF may act on hepatocyte proliferation less effectively in damaged liver than in normal liver. Such deficiency of the stimulatory activity in damaged liver might be a cause of insufficient liver regeneration in patients with fulminant hepatic failure.

References

1. O'Grady JC, Portman B, Williams R. In: Schiff L et al (eds) Diseases of the Liver, 7th edn. Philadelphia: Lippincal Company, 1993;1077–1090.
2. Popper H, Keppler D. In: Popper H, Schaffner F (eds) Progress in Liver Disease, vol 8. Oriando: Grune and Stratton, 1966;209–235.
3. Esmon CT. J Biol Chem 1989;264:4743–4746.
4. Car BD, Slauson DO, Suyemoto MM et al. Exp Lung Res 1991;17:939–957.
5. Geczy CL, Farram E, Moon DK et al. J Immunol 1983;130:2743–2749.
6. Conkling PR, Greenberg CS, Weinberg JB. Blood 1988;72:128–133.
7. Nemerson Y. Blood 1988;71:1–8.
8. Takano S, Kimura S, Ohdama S et al. Blood 1990;76:2024–2029.
9. Arai M, Mochida S, Ohno A et al. Thrombosis Res Coagulibility in rat liver microcirculation as evaluated by endothelial cell modulation and macrophage tissue factor. (in press).
10. Arai M, Mochida S, Ohno A et al. Transplant Proc 1994;26:913–915.
11. Mochida S, Ohno A, Arai M et al. Hepatology 1994; 20:182A.
12. Hische EAH, Tutuarima JA, van der Helm HJ. Clin Chem 1981;27:1427–1430.
13. Fujiwara K, Ogata I, Ohta Y et al. Gut 1988;29:1103–1108.
14. Hirata K, Ogata I, Ohta Y et al. J Pathol 1989;158:157–165.
15. Ferluga J, Allison AC. Lancet 1978;2:610–611.
16. Mochida S, Ogata I, Hirata K et al. Gastroenterology 1990;99:771–777.
17. Fujiwara K, Ogata I, Mochida S et al. Hepato-Gastroenterol 1990;37:194–197.
18. Ogata I, Mochida S, Fujiwara K. Biomed Res 1988;9:113–117.
19. Mochida S, Ogata I, Ohta Y et al. J Pathol 1989;158:67–71.
20. Mochida S, Masaki N, Ohta Y et al. J Pathol 1992;167:83–89.
21. Mochida S, Ohta Y, Ogata I et al. J Hepatol 1992;16:266–272.
22. Fujiwara K, Mochida S, Nagoshi S et al. J Ethinopharmacol Regulation of hepatic macrophage function by oral administration of Xiao-Chai-Hu-Tang (Sho-Saiko-To, TJ-9) in rats. (in press).
23. Yamada S, Ogata I, Hirata K et al. Scand J Gastroenterol 1989;24:293–298.
24. Arai M, Mochida S, Ohno A et al. Gastroenterology 1993;104:1466–1471.
25. Mochida S, Arai M, Ohno A et al. Liver 1994;14:234–240.
26. Ohno A, Mochida S, Arai M et al. Dig Dis Sci 1994;39:861–865.
27. Arai M, Mochida S, Ohno A et al. Hepatology 1994;20:198A.
28. Fujiwara K, Nagoshi S, Ohno A et al. Hepatology 1993;18:1443–1449.
29. Sato Y, Fujiwara K. J Biochem 1988;104:98–101.
30. Pegg AE, Matsui I, Seely JE et al. Med Biol 1981;59:327–333.
31. Nagoshi S, Fujiwara K. Hepatology 1994;20:725–730.

32. Nakamura T, Yoshimoto K, Nakayama Y et al. Proc Natl Acad Sci USA 1983;80:7229–7233.
33. Yamada S, Fujiwara K, Oka Y et al. J Biochem 1986;101:1385–1389.
34. Hirata K, Fujiwara K. Biochem Biophys Res Commun 1990;171:1093–1098.
35. Hirata K, Fujiwara K. Biomed Res 1991;12:425–428.
36. Tomiya T, Nagoshi S, Fujiwara K. Hepatology 1992;15:1–4.
37. Tomiya T, Yani M, Yamada S et al. Gastroenterology 1992;103:1621–1624.
38. Tomiya T, Fujiwara K. Hepatology 1993;18:304–308.
39. Tomiya T, Hirata K, Ikeda K et al. Hepatology 1994;20:222A.
40. Tomiya T, Fujiwara K. Hepatology 1993;18:195A.

Progress in Hepatology Vol. 1.
Cellular and Molecular Biology.
M. Yamanaka, K. Okabe and G. Toda, editors.

The effect of HGF on coagulation and fibrinolysis in dimethylnitrosoamine-induced liver injury

Kazuhiko Okabe,[1] Hiroshi Suzuki,[1] Yukio Kato,[1] Michihiro Suzuki,[1] Shoichi Suemori[1] and Takashi Meguro[2]

[1]Internal Medicine, and [2]Division of Research Laboratory, St Marianna University School of Medicine, Yokohama City Seibu Hospital, Yokohama 241, Japan

Abstract. Recent studies have demonstrated that a strong secondary tissue plasminagen activator (t-PA) activity may occur locally in the liver followed by enhanced fibrinolysis in particular in fulminant hepatitis and hepatic cirrhosis. In this study with a rat experiment, it was observed that the dimethylnitrosamine (DMN)-induced hepatic injury showed elevations in both AST and alanine aminotransferase (ALT), decreases in total protein, coagulation activity such as NT and platelet count. The administration of t-PA to this DMN-induced liver injury gave rise to intensive abnormalities in laboratory findings such as AST, ALT, and the coagulation system and in histological findings. Also survival was extremely low compared with the DMN group. These results suggest coagulofibrinolysis abnormalities strongly aggravate liver damage. On the other hand, the tumor cytotoxic factor (TCF), a kind of hepatocyte growth factor (HGF), which is a 5-amino acid residue deleted type at the domain corresponding to the first kringle (a deletion variant of HGF, dHGF), apparently suppressed both the DMN- and the DMN plus t-PA-induced hepatopathy. TCF administration showed a remarkable improvement in both laboratory and pathological findings, and the protective and regenerative effects of TCF on hepatocytes have been confirmed.

Key words: coagulofibrinolysis, dimethylnitrosoamine-induced liver injury, hepatocyte growth factor, liver disease, tissue plasminogen activator, transforming growth factor-β.

Introduction

Coagulation and fibrinolytic patterns in liver disease show various changes together with the vicissitudes of the disease [1–5]. Our clinical data show decreases in production of fibrinogen, plasminogen, vitamin K-dependent factors (factors II, VII, IX and X) and antithrombin-III (AT-III), α_2-plasmin inhibitor (α_2-PI) in liver diseases [6–8]. Further, platelets generate adhesion and aggregation in the liver reticular system and a decrease was observed

Address for correspondence: Kazuhiko Okabe, M.D., Internal Medicine St Marianna University School of Medicine, Yokohama City Seibu Hospital, 1197-1 Yazashi-Cyo, Yokohama 241, Japan. Tel: +81-45-366-1111.

through consumption or pooling in the spleen. In particular, the enhancement of the coagulation and fibrinolytic system in fulminant hepatitis and hepatic cirrhosis is a phenomenon corresponding to disseminated intravascular coagulation (DIC) or pre-DIC, in which mild to severe hepatic local changes in the balance of tissue plasminogen activator (t-PA) and t-PA inhibitor-1 (PAI-1) are presumed to be involved. Coagulation and fibrinolytic abnormalities induce liver damage and produce a hepatocyte growth factor (HGF) [9–11] from Kupffer cells, Ito cells and sinusoidal endothelial cells to keep the tissue homeostasis.

In this study, we attempted to elucidate the role of the coagulofibrinolysis in hepatic damage both clinically and experimentally and also the effect of HGF in experimental liver injury.

Materials and Methods

The patients were 53 cases with liver cirrhosis (31 compensated hepatic cirrhosis; 22 decompensated hepatic cirrhosis) who have visited our hospital since 1988, while 10 healthy adults were used as normal controls. Blood was taken early in the morning while fasting and EDTA blood was used for measurements of red blood cell (rbc), leucocyte, platelet counts and Hb concentration. The measurements of blood coagulation and fibrinolytic factors were made on 1/10 vol. 3.8% sodium citrated plasma stored at −80°C until the assay.

Fisher strain male rats were used. In order to lessen the variations during experiments, rats were kept in cages of four each and fed a normal diet. Rats of 6 weeks of age were acclimatized for 1 week before the start of the experiment. Three groups of rats were prepared. The first group of 4 rats had dimethylnitrosamine (DMN) damage (DMN), the second group of 8 rats were used to observe the additional effects of tissue plasminogen activator (t-PA) (DMN + t-PA), the third group of 4 rats were used to observe the effect of hepatocyte growth factor (HGF) on the first group (DMN + TCF), and the fourth group of 8 rats were used to observe the effects of HGF on the second group (DMN + TCF + t-PA). The normal control group had 8 nontreated rats of 11 weeks of age.

DMN JIS-GR (Wako Pure Chemical Industries, Ltd.) with a molecular weight of 74.08 and specific gravity of 1.010 was used. The DMN solution for injection was prepared before use as a 10 μg/ml concentration (100-fold dilution of DMN) with physiological saline (Otsuka Pharmaceutical Co., Ltd.) and given at a dose of 10 μg/kg intraperitoneally every other day, 3 times a week [12].

For HGF, 5-amino acid residue-deleted-type recombinant TCF (Biological Science Laboratory, Snow Brand Milk Products Co., Ltd.) [13,14] was used. The potency of the HGF (TCF) solution was assayed by rat hepatocyte DNA

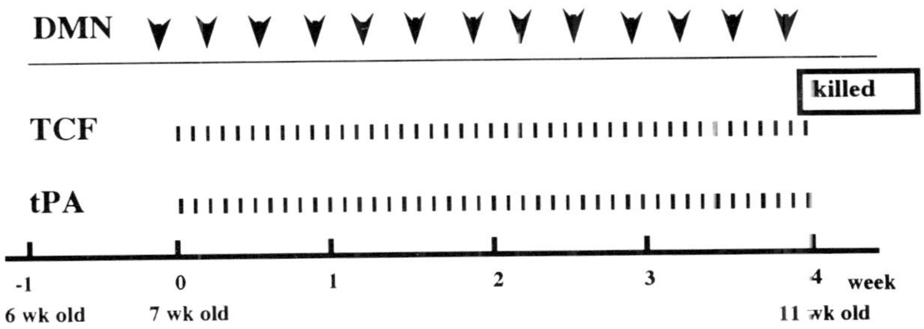

Fig. 1. Experimental schedule in rats with DMN-induced liver injury.

synthesis, and a 500 μg/ml solution (HGF vehicle solution, frozen at -80°C) was prepared. The frozen solution was thawed at 37°C before use, and 500 μg/kg/dose was injected intravenously into the tail vein twice a day in the morning and evening. In addition, as the control for HGF, the vehicle of TCF was similarly injected.

For t-PA, a recombinant product, 6 million units of GLUTOPA t-PA (Mitsubishi Kasei Corporation) was used. Six million units of t-PA were dissolved in 10 ml of physiological saline (600,000 units/ml) and frozen at -80°C. It was thawed just before use, diluted to 75,000 units/ml, and 250,000 units/kg was intravenously injected through the tail vein twice a day, in the morning and evening (Fig. 1).

Rats were laparotomied under ethylether (Wako Pure Chemical Industries, Ltd) anesthesia and using a 22 G needle, 5 ml of 1/10 volume 3.8% sodium citrated blood and 1 ml of blood to which EDTA-2K was added were taken from the inferior vena cava. The plasma (sodium citrated plasma) obtained by centrifugation at 3,000 rpm for 15 minutes, was subjected to the blood chemical analysis and assay of coagulation and fibrinolytic systems. The blood to which EDTA-2K had been added was used for the measurement of platelets, red blood cells (RBC), white blood cells (WBC) and hemaglobin (Hb). Immediately after blood sampling, tissues of the liver and spleen were taken out, followed by formalin fixation and liquid nitrogen freezing, and subjected to the histopathological examination. The liver was lavaged with physiological saline from the portal vein, frozen, and used for assays of liver hydroxyproline and TGF-β.

D-dimer, t-PA, t-PA inhibitor-1 (PAI-1), plasminogen, α_2-plasmin inhibitor (α_2-PI), plasminogen-α_2-PI complex (PIC), thrombin-antithrombin III complex (TAT) were assayed by the EIA method. Normotest (NT, Eisai Co., Ltd.) was made by the addition of 10 μl of 2$\times$ diluted plasma to 250 μl of NT reagent and assay with KC-10 (Baxter), and the activity (%) was obtained from the standard curve. The activity of factor VIII was assayed by additions of 100 μl of a pathromtin reagent (PTT, Behring) and 100 μl of 25 mM $CaCl_2$ to 100 μl of factor VIII-deficient human plasma (reagent for the determination of coagulation Factor VIII, Behring) and 100 μl of diluted plasma and with KC-10 (Baxter). Fibrinogen was determined by the addition of 5× diluted plasma to 200 μl of thrombin reagent (Hitothrombin, Ortho) and with KC-10. Antithrombin III (AT-III) activity and α_2-PI activity were assayed by an endpoint assay using synthesized substrates for AT-III and α_2-PI.

AST and ALT were determined by the UV method (autoanalyzer HR2400, JEOL Ltd.) and total protein by the Biuret method.

For determination of the liver hydroxyproline, rat liver (500 mg) was homogenized in Folch solution, followed by filtration by suction to remove fat completely and completely dehydrated with methanol and ether, and a dry powder was prepared. The dry powder (10 mg) was taken in a 2 ml-capped tube, 1 ml of 6 N HCl was added, the tube was tightly closed, and after hydrolysis at 107°C for 16 hours, the HCl was thoroughly removed in a rotary evaporator and the volume was made up to 1 ml with distilled water. The extracted sample (200 μl) was mixed with 200 ml of chloramine T solution and was allowed to stand still at room temperature for 20 minutes, 200 μl of aldehyde/perchloric acid solution was added and the solution mixed well. After warming at 60°C for 15 minutes, it was immediately cooled and assayed with an absorption spectrophotometer at 550 nm. The amount of hydroxyproline was obtained from a standard curve prepared with L-hydroxyproline (Tokyo Kasei).

For determination of the liver TGF-β, total TGF-β (both active and inactive forms) was isolated from the plasma by acid-methanol extraction. Because this extraction procedure activates TGF-β, we could not determine the amount of active and inactive TGF-β present in the samples. To extract TGF-β, 3 ml of an acid-methanol solution (50% methanol/10 mM HCl/1 mM phenylmethylsulfonyl fluoride) was added to 0.5 g liver tissue. The liver tissue was homogenized with a Potter homogenizer. The homogenate was stirred overnight at 4°C, then centrifuged at 12,000 g for 30 minutes at 4°C. The supernatant was dialyzed overnight against 1 M acetic acid, divided into aliquots, lyophilized, and stored at −20°C. The extracted samples were reconstituted in 5 mM HCl containing 0.1% bovine serum albumin before assay. The evaluation of the TGF-β content of the samples was performed using a commercially available TGF-β ELISA kit (Amersham Co.).

From the histopathological examination, hematoxylin-eosin stain, Masson's trichrome stain and silver stain were performed. Identification of antiproliferating cell nuclear antigen (PCNA) was attempted using a PCNA mouse monoclonal antibody (DAKO-PCNA, PC-10), stained by avidinbiotin-complex method (ABC method) and the number of PCNA-positive cell nuclei/1,000 of liver cell nuclei was obtained.

For the statistical analysis, Bonferroni's method was used, and the level of significance was assigned as $p < 0.05$.

Results

Coagulation and fibrinolytic factors in hepatic cirrhosis

In compensated hepatic cirrhosis, the platelet count was $98 \pm 31 \times 10^3/mm^3$ (n = 26) and plasminogen was 74.2 ± 12.1% (n = 24), while in the decompensated hepatic cirrhosis group, platelet count was $76 \pm 5 \times 10^3/mm^3$ (n = 7) and plasminogen was 51.4 ± 6.5% (n = 5), which was respectively significantly ($p < 0.05$) low.

In the compensated hepatic cirrhosis group, NT was 66.7 ± 13.8% (n = 24), AT-III was 66.0 ± 12.4% (n = 24), fibrinogen was 168.5 ± 42.8 mg/dl (n = 24), α_2-PI was 64.7 ± 11.4%, while in the decompensated hepatic cirrhosis, they were 58.9 ± 14.4% (n = 7), 55.9 ± 23.3% (n = 7), 186.0 ± 40.9 mg/dl (n = 7), 51.4 ± 22.1% (n = 7), respectively, showing low values as compared with normal controls, but there was no significant difference between the two groups. In compensated cirrhosis, TAT was 6.3 ± 10.9 μg/ml (n = 32) and PIC was 0.98 ± 0.64 μg/ml (n = 34), while in the decompensated cirrhosis group, they were 13.4 ± 15.7 μg/ml (n = 7) and 0.81 ± 0.74 μg/ml (n = 14), respectively, showing no significant difference between the two groups. However, TAT was significantly high ($p < 0.05$) as compared with the value in healthy adults. In compensated hepatic cirrhosis, t-PA was 10.8 ± 5.8 ng/ml (n = 31) and in the decompensated hepatic cirrhosis, it was 21.6 ± 10.4 ng/ml (n = 22), significantly higher ($p < 0.05$) compared with both compensated hepatic cirrhosis and 5.6 ± 2.5 ng/ml (n = 10) of normal controls. Further, in the compensated hepatic cirrhosis, PAI-1 was 23.4 ± 12.8 ng/ml (n = 28), and 27.4 ± 6.4 ng/ml (n = 14) in the decompensated hepatic cirrhosis, both of them were significantly high ($p < 0.05$) as compared with 13.6 ± 6.7 ng/ml (n = 10) of the healthy adults (Table 1). Further, hepatic cirrhosis was divided into four groups (A, B, C and D) according to the degree of changes in fibrinolytic parameters. In the compensated hepatic cirrhosis group, there was 1 (2.8%) in the A group (t-PA: >11 ng/ml and PAI-1: >14 ng/ml), 0 in the B group (t-PA: ≤11 ng/ml and PAI-1: >14 ng/ml), and there were 17 each (48.6%) in the C group

Table 1. Correlation between t-PA and PAI-1 in liver cirrhosis

	t-PA(ng/ml)	PAI-1(ng/ml)	t-PA/PAI-1 ratio(%)
Control	5.6 ± 2.5 (n = 10)	13.3 ± 6.9 (n = 9)	53.3 ± 34.4 (n = 9)
Compensated hepatic cirrhosis	10.8 ± 5.8 (n = 31)**	23.4 ± 12.8 (n = 28)*	50.0 ± 19.3 (n = 28)
Decompensated hepatic cirrhosis	21.6 ± 10.4 (n = 22)**	27.4 ± 6.4 (n = 14)**	82.8 ± 28.7 (n = 14)**

*$p < 0.05$; **$p < 0.01$.

(t-PA: ≤11 ng/ml and PAI-1: ≤14 ng/ml) and the D group (t-PA: >11 ng/ml and PAI-1: ≤14 ng/ml), while in the decompensated hepatic cirrhosis, there were 2 (15.3%), 1 (7.7%), 3 (23%) and 7 (53.8%) respectively, showing differences between the compensated and decompensated groups. Furthermore, the t-PA:PAI-1 ratio (%) was 50.0 ± 19.3% (n = 28) in the compensated hepatic cirrhosis group, 82.8 ± 28.7% (n = 28) in decompensated hepatic cirrhosis, showing a significantly high value ($p < 0.05$) in the latter, even compared with the value in healthy adults of 53.3 ± 34.4% (n = 9). The t-PA of decompensated hepatic cirrhosis was about 1.7× higher than that of compensated hepatic cirrhosis and normal adults. Cases with D-dimer >500 ng/ml accounted for 16% of compensated hepatic cirrhosis and 43% of decompensated hepatic cirrhosis. In particular, 8% of compensated hepatic cirrhosis cases and 36% of decompensated hepatic cirrhosis cases, had t-PA >11 ng/ml and D-dimer >500 ng/ml indicating that decompensated cases were in a significantly more enhanced fibrinolytic state than the former ($p < 0.05$).

The effects of t-PA and HGF in DMN-induced liver injuries

After giving 0, 10, 100 and 1,000 μg/kg/day of TCF, the values of markers such as total protein, serum albumin and platelet count suggested that 1,000 μg/kg/day of TCF was the optimal dose (Fig. 2).

The survival rates of the DMN group (n = 4) and the DMN + TCF group (n = 4) were 100%. However, in the group given t-PA, 10 of 16 (62.5%) died after 25 days. That is, the survival rate of the DMN + t-PA group (n = 8) was 13% (7 died), and that of the DMN + t-PA + TCF group (n = 8) was 63% (only 3 died). The survival rate of the DMN + t-PA group (n = 8) significantly ($p < 0.01$) decreased in comparison with the TCF-treated group. The survival rate of the DMN + t-PA group given TCF (DMN + t-PA + TCF) showed an apparent ($p < 0.01$) improvement effect in comparison with that of the DMN + t-PA group (Table 2).

Table 2. Effects of TCF, t-PA administration on survival rate in rats with DMN-induced liver injury

	Rats	Died	Survived	Survival rate (%)
Normal control	8	0	8	100
DMN + vehicle of TCF	4	0	4	100
DMN + TCF	4	0	4	100
DMN + t-PA	8	7	1	13
DMN + t-PA + TCF	8	3	5	63

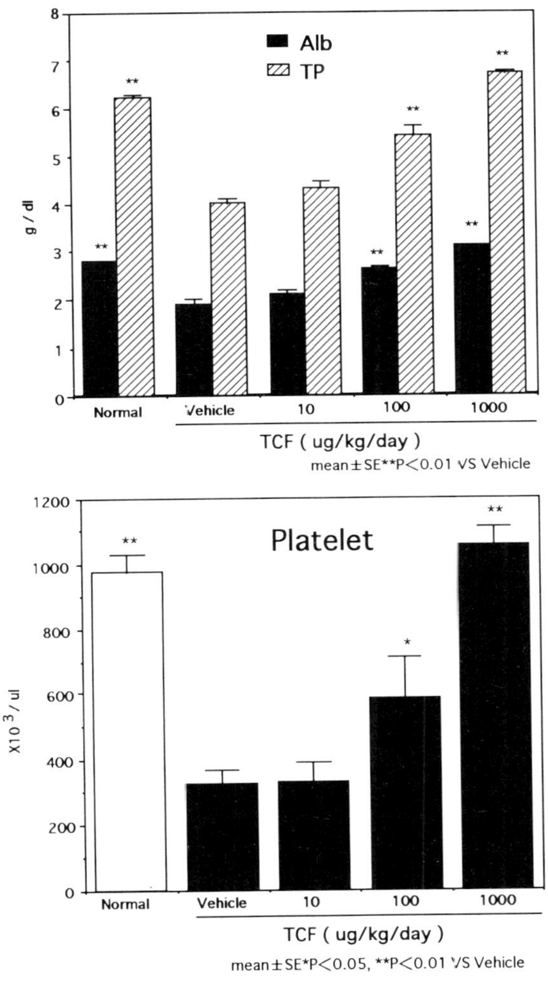

Fig. 2. Effect of various doses of TCF on serum albumin, total protein and peripheral blood platelets levels in rats with DMN-induced liver injury.

Laboratory findings

RBC and platelet count (Fig. 3). The DMN-induced liver injury group (DMN group) showed an RBC count of $6560 + 165 \times 10^3/\mu l$ (n = 4) and a platelet count of $93 \pm 40 \times 10^3/\mu l$ (n = 4), which were significantly ($p<0.01$) low compared with those of the normal group [RBC $9{,}114 \pm 108 \times 10^3/\mu l$ (n = 7), platelet count $727 \pm 18 \times 10^3/\mu l$ (n = 7)]. The DMN + t-PA group showed an RBC of $2{,}900 \times 10^3/\mu l$ (n = 1) and a platelet count of $33 \times 10^3/\mu l$ (n = 1); both of them were markedly ($p<0.01$) low, compared with the DMN group.

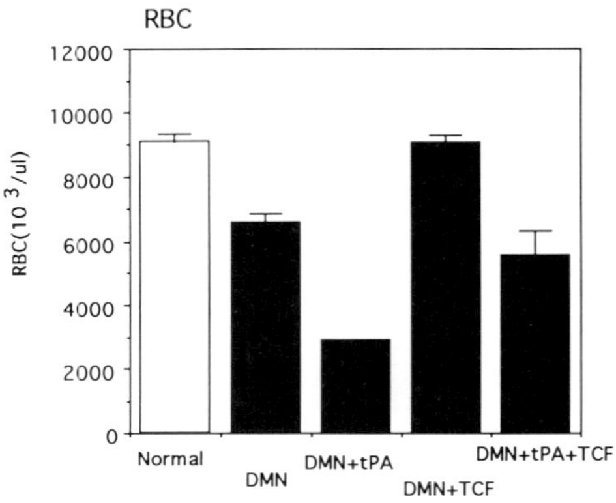

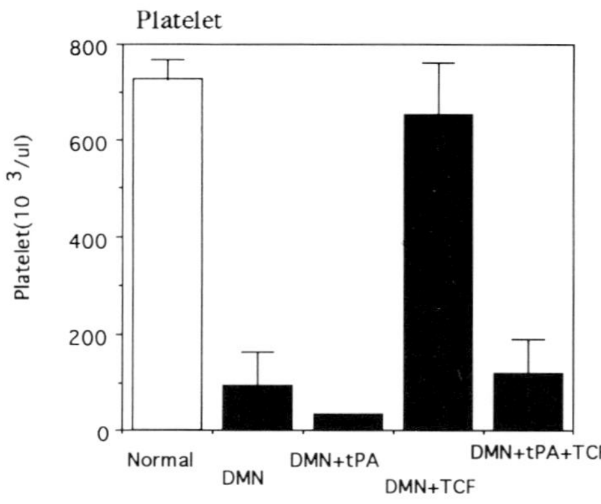

Fig. 3. Effects of TCF, t-PA administration on peripheral blood RBC, and platelets levels in rats with DMN-induced liver injury.

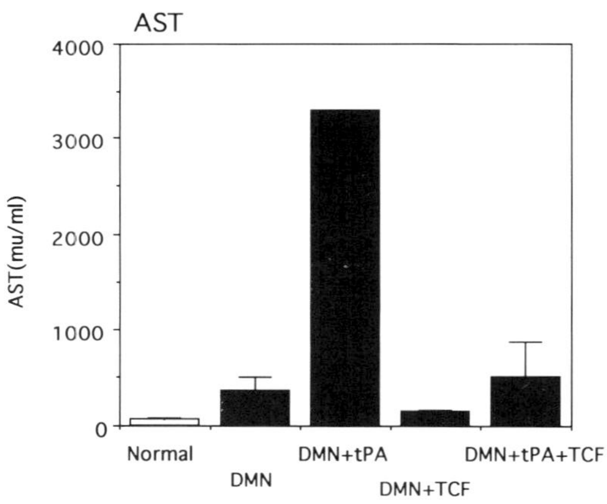

Fig. 4. Effects of TCF, t-PA administration on serum AST level in rats with DMN-induced liver injury.

The DMN group given TCF showed an RBC of $9{,}068 \pm 127 \times 10^3/\mu l$ and a platelet count of $65 \pm 54 \times 10^3/\mu l$, which did not differ from the normal group, suggesting an improvement due to the TCF administration. The DMN + t-PA + TCF group showed an RBC of $5{,}532 \pm 338 \times 10^3/\mu l$ and a platelet count of $119 \pm 31 \times 10^3/\mu l$, which were not improved to the level of the normal group, but showed significant ($p < 0.01$) improvement by the TCF administration in comparison with the DMN + t-PA group.

AST (Fig. 4). The DMN group showed AST of 350.8 ± 147.2 μ/ml, which was a significantly ($p < 0.05$) elevated in comparison with the normal group of

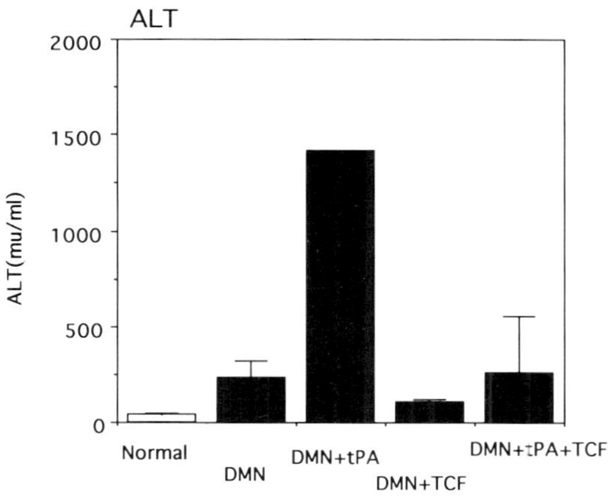

Fig. 5. Effects of TCF, t-PA administration on serum ALT level in rats with DMN-induced liver injury.

69.4 ± 8.7 μ/ml. Further, the DMN + t-PA group was 3,294 μ/ml markedly high ($p < 0.01$) in comparison with the normal and DMN groups. As to the effects of TCF, the DMN + TCF and DMN + t-PA + TCF groups showed 141.5 ± 19.3 μ/ml and 499.0 ± 364.9 μ/ml, respectively, which were higher than the normal group, but significantly ($p < 0.01$) lower than the groups without TCF, indicating a favorable effect of TCF administration.

ALT (Fig. 5). The changes of ALT were approximately the same as those of AST, such as 235.3 ± 89.2 μ/ml (n = 4) and 1,413 μ/ml (n = 1) in the DMN and DMN + t-PA groups, respectively, showing significant ($p < 0.05$) elevations in comparison with 38.3 ± 8.8 mu/ml of the normal group. Further, the DMN + t-PA group showed a significantly ($p < 0.01$) higher value even than that of the DMN group. The DMN + TCF and DMN + t-PA + TCF groups showed 108.3 ± 9.9 μ/ml (n = 4) and 260.2 ± 296.0 μ/ml (n = 5), respectively, showing significant ($p < 0.01$) improvement with the administration of TCF.

Total protein in plasma (Fig. 6). In comparison with the value of 5.16 ± 0.10 g/dl (n = 7) in the normal group, the DMN group showed a significant ($p < 0.01$) decrease to 4.00 ± 0.29 g/dl (n = 4). Furthermore, the value in the DMN + t-PA group decreased significantly ($p < 0.01$) to 2.10 g/dl (n = 1) compared with that of the DMN group. The DMN + TCF group showed 4.93 ± 0.33 g/dl (n = 4) and the DMN + t-PA + TCF group showed 3.62 ± 0.13 g/dl (n = 5), which were significantly ($p < 0.01$) improved as compared with the DMN and DMN + t-PA groups.

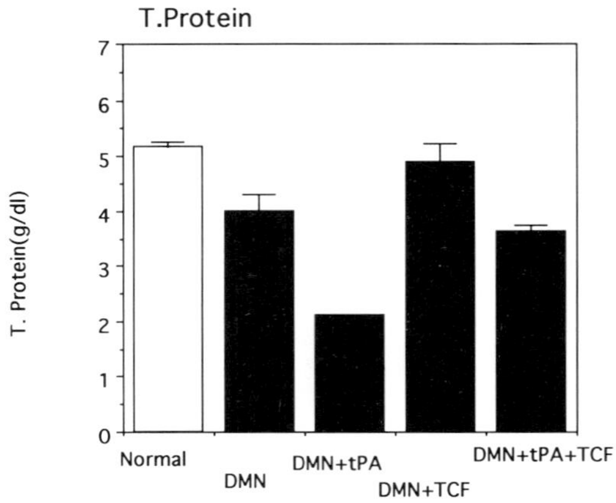

Fig. 6. Effects of TCF, t-PA administration on serum protein level in rats with DMN-induced liver injury.

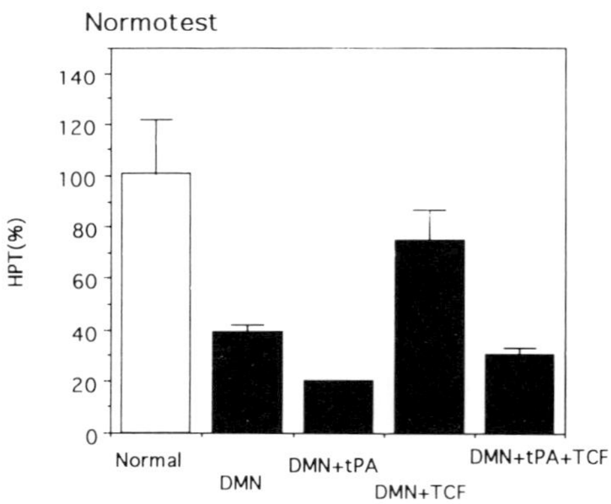

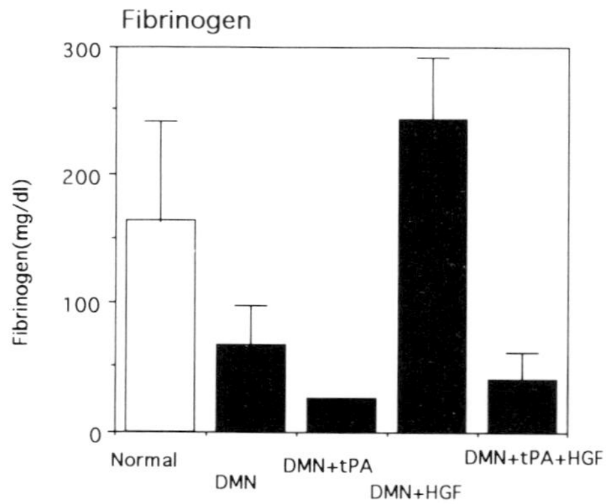

Fig. 7. Effects of TCF, t-PA administration on normotest and fibrinogen in rats with DMN-induced liver injury.

NT and fibrinogen (Fig. 7). The DMN group showed NT of $39 \pm 1.3\%$ ($n = 4$) and fibrinogen of 67 ± 16 mg/dl ($n = 4$), which were significantly ($p < 0.01$ and $p < 0.05$) lower than those in the normal group with NT of $100 \pm 8.5\%$ ($n = 7$) and fibrinogen of 163 ± 29 mg/dl ($n = 7$). The DMN + t-PA group was as significantly ($p < 0.01$) low [NT of 25% ($n = 1$) and fibrinogen of 35 mg/dl ($n = 1$)]. The DMN + TCF group showed NT of $75 \pm 5.9\%$ ($n = 4$) and fibrinogen of 243 ± 25 mg/dl ($n = 4$), which were similar to values in the normal group, however, in comparison with the DMN group, significant increases in NT ($p < 0.05$) and fibrinogen ($p < 0.01$) were observed. In the DMN + t-PA + TCF group, NT was 30 ± 1.5%, which was not significantly different from both the DMN and DMN + t-PA groups and fibrinogen was 450 ± 9.3 mg/dl showing rather higher than normal and DMN + TCF groups.

Factor VIII. The DMN group showed 87 ± 15% (n = 4), which was not significantly different from 100% of the normal group, while the DMN + t-PA group showed a marked ($p < 0.01$) decrease to 10% (n = 1). The DMN + TCF group was 108 ± 7% (n = 4), while the DMN + t-PA + TCF group was 20 ± 10%, without any significant improvement.

α_2-PI and AT-III. In the DMN-induced liver injury group, α_2-PI was 67 ± 5% and AT-III was 200 ± 15%, which were not significantly different from α_2-PI of 75 ± 20% and AT-III of 100% in the normal group. However, in the DMN + t-PA group, they markedly ($p < 0.01$) decreased to α_2-PI of 10% and AT-III of 10%. The DMN + TCF group showed significant ($p < 0.01$) increases to α_2-PI of 94 ± 15% and AT-III of 500 ± 120%. The DMN + t-PA + TCF group also markedly increased to an α_2-PI of 70 ± 10% and AT-III of 45 ± 10% in comparison with DMN + t-PA group; however it did not recover to the level of the normal group.

Liver hydroxyproline. The hydroxyproline value of the DMN-induced liver injury group was 7.8 ± 1.5 μ/mg defatted dry wt. (n = 4) which was significantly ($p < 0.01$) higher than the 3.32 ± 0.72 μg/mg defatted dry wt. of the normal group. The DMN + t-PA group showed 22.77 μg/mg defatted dry wt. (n = 1), which was significantly ($p < 0.01$) higher than the DMN group. The DMN + TCF group showed a trend towards improvement, (5.95 ± 0.061 μg/mg defatted dry wt., n = 4). The DMN + t-PA + TCF group showed 12.99 ± 5.60 μg/ml (n = 8), which was a significant ($p < 0.05$) decrease compared with the DMN + t-PA group.

Liver TGF-β. In the DMN-induced liver injury group there was TGF-β of 2.77 ± 0.19 ng/g wet tissue, which was higher than the 1.56 ± 0.15 ng/g wet tissue of the normal group. The DMN + t-PA + TCF group showed only 1.00 ng/g wet tissue (n = 1). The DMN + TCF group (n = 4) showed 1.77 ± 0.60 ng/g wet tissue, indicating a trend towards improvement.

Histopathological findings

The centrilobular area of the liver of the DMN group showed hemorrhagic necrosis on hematoxylin-eosine (HE) stain (Fig. 8A). Slight perilobular infiltrations of lymphocytes and granulocytes were observed, and an apparent increase of collagen was observed at centrilobular necrotic lesion and periportal area. On silver stain (Fig. 9A), the centrilobular area was deciduated and the condensation of the reticulin fiber was prominent with marked bridging formation. On PCNA stain (Fig. 10A), PCNA-positive hepatocyte nuclei were sporadically observed, so that slight liver tissue repair was suggested. The centrilobular area of the DMN + t-PA group (n = 1) showed a ballooning necrosis, and deciduation, hemorrhage and edema of hepatocytes were observed, which were more severe than those in the DMN group, the perilobular area was nodular and the basophillity of the hepatocytes was not retained. Furthermore, there was neither nuclear mytosis nor recruitment of Kupffer cells (Fig. 8B). On silver stain (Fig. 9B), almost no fiber formation was observed, but intense edema was observed at the centrilobular area with liquefaction and rupture, and no condensation of reticulin fiber was observed in magnified fields (×100). In PCNA stain (Fig. 10B), no increase of the PCNA-positive hepatocytes was observed and the reparation of the liver tissue was poor. The centrilobular area of the DMN + TCF group did not show any hemorrhagic necrosis, only slight edema in parts. Nuclear mytosis was sporadically seen at the interlobular area and the DMN-induced liver injury was apparently suppressed, suggesting repair of the liver damage (Fig. 8C). In silver stain (Fig. 9C), there was almost no fibroplasia and general condensation of reticulin and on PCNA stain (Fig. 10C), the proliferation of PCNA-positive hepatocyte was apparently observed compared with the DMN group. The centrilobular area of the DMN + t-PA + TCF group showed some hemorrhagic spots, but there was no deciduation or edema and no mytosis was observed, showing an apparent suppression of liver injury (Fig. 8D). In silver stain (Fig. 9D), a little condensation of reticulin fiber was observed, but the proliferation of PCNA-positive hepatocytes was much more common than in the DMN + t-PA group (Fig. 10D).

Discussion

The changes of the coagulation and fibrinolytic system are observed in various liver diseases [1–5]. In fulminant hepatitis and advanced hepatic cirrhosis, coagulofibrinolytic factors and inhibitors are triggered by platelets trapped in the liver reticular system, and the activation of the coagulation system is in accordance with a decrease of plasminogen, α_2-PI and an increase of PAI-1. It suggests that a strong secondary t-PA activity may occur locally in the liver, followed by enhanced fibrinolysis.

In this study, it was observed that in rats, the DMN-induced hepatic injury showed elevations in both AST and ALT, and decreases in total protein, coagulation activity such as NT and platelet count.

The administration of t-PA to this DMN-induced liver injury gave rise to intensive abnormalities in both AST and ALT and the coagulation system. In this group survival was extremely low compared with the DMN group.

The facts strongly indicate that t-PA aggravates the liver damage as we have reported previously [8]. Clinically, the mechanism of aggravating liver

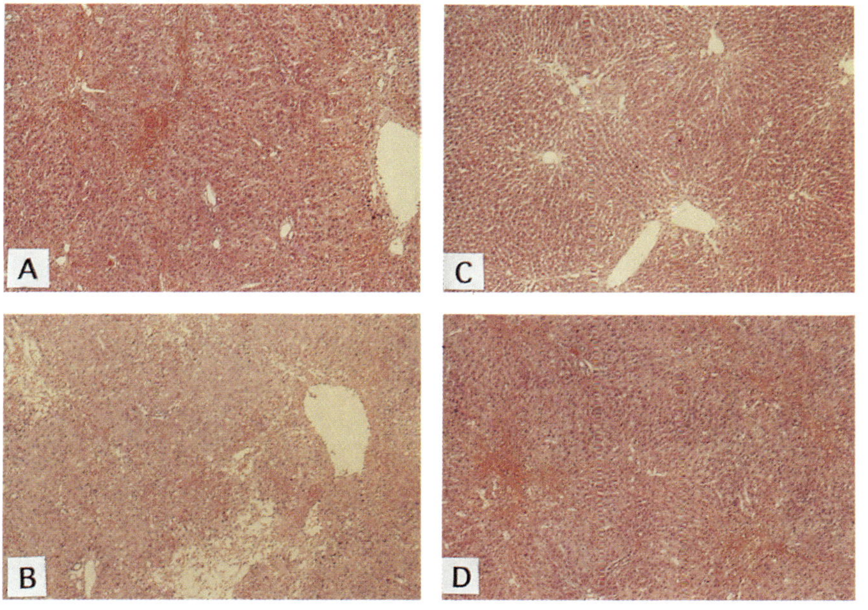

Fig. 8. Histological changes of the liver from a rat with DMN-induced liver injury. Each group shows HE stain (100×). A: no administration of t-PA or TCF. B: administration of t-PA. C: administration of TCF. D: administration of t-PA and TCF.

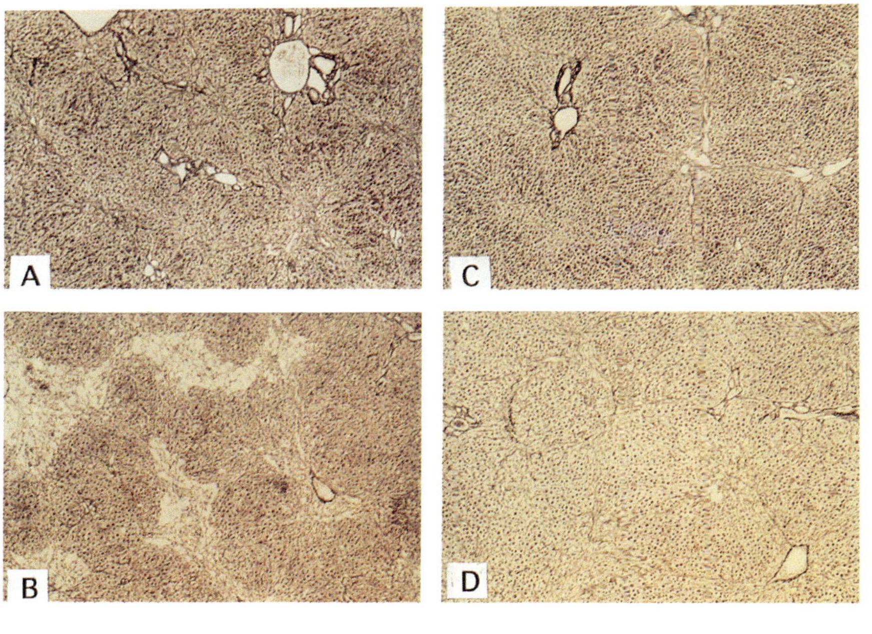

Fig. 9. Histological changes of the liver from a rat with DMN-induced liver injury. Each group shows silver stain (100×). A: no administration of t-PA or TCF. B: administration of t-PA. C: administration of TCF. D: administration of t-PA and TCF.

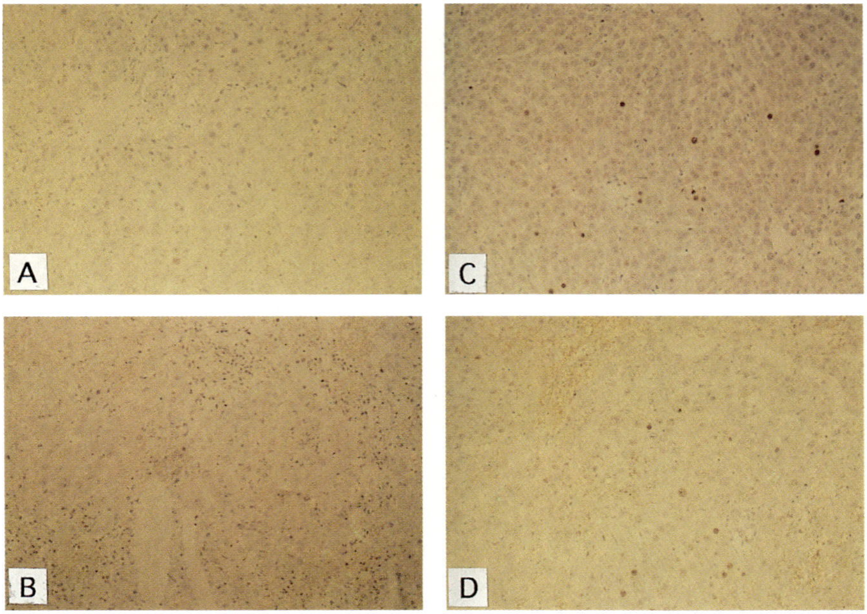

Fig. 10. Histological changes of the liver from a rat with DMN-induced liver injury. Each group shows PCNA stain (200×). A: no administration of t-PA or TCF. B: administration of t-PA. C: administration of TCF. D: administration of t-PA and TCF.

damage mediated by the fibrinolytic system is unknown, however, one possibility is that the proliferation of nonparenchymal cells such as Ito cells in the damaged liver may accelerate the release of intrinsic HGF [10,11] and TGF-β [15,16]. It was thought that HGF acts on promotion of hepatocyte proliferation to regenerate the liver, while TGF-β acts suppressively, thus the homeostasis of tissue regeneration and wound healing for the liver damage is maintained. However, HGF and TGF-β have various biological activities, and are involved with the fibrinolytic system. HGF stimulates sinusoidal endothelial cells in the liver tissue and promotes the release of t-PA and u-PA to produce fibrinolysis [17–20]. Further, it releases TGF-β which stimulates the release of PAI-1, and inhibits t-PA activity to maintain homeostasis in the liver tissue [21,22].

The TCF used in this study is a kind of HGF, which is a 5-amino acid residue-deleted type at the domain corresponding to the first kringle (a deletion variant of HGF, dHGF) and its biological activity is somewhat different from the conventional HGF. Particularly, in an in vitro cell culture system, the conventional HGF shows a maximum activity at 10 ng/ml and the activity rapidly decreases at higher concentrations, while TCF keeps its maximum activity throughout the range 10–100 ng/ml, and the specific activity is also high [13]. When TCF was consecutively given to normal and hepatectomized rats, increase of liver weight and elevation in puretoscine and putrescine which are enzymes that accelerate DNA synthesis have been confirmed.

The effects of HGF have been reported in vivo on partial hepatectomized and drug-induced liver damage animals and in in vitro cultured cells also [23–25]. However, most reports were performed with acute hepatic damage and little has been reported on chronic hepatic damage. In this paper, we have used TCF consecutively for 4 weeks in rats. As regards pathological findings, t-PA was remarkably aggravated in rats with DMN-induced liver injury.

TCF apparently suppressed the DMN and DMN plus t-PA-induced hepatopathy from both laboratory and histological standpoints.

Increased TGF-β content in the liver may be involved in liver damage through collagen formation. Thus, it was supposed that the production of collagen mediated by Ito cells, as well as inhibition of collagenase production and acceleration of tissue inhibitor of metaloprotenase (TIMP) production were involved [26, 27].

References

1. Booth NA, Anderson JA et al. J Clin Pathol 1984;37:772–777.
2. Kashiwabara T, Takikawa Y et al. Blood and Vessel 1985;16:629–632.
3. Rake MO, Flute PT et al. Lancet 1970;1:533–537.
4. Verstraete M, Vermylen J et al. Ann Rev Med 1974;25:447–455.
5. Rake MO, Flute PT et al. Lancet 1971;II:1215–1218.
6. Okabe K, Kato I et al. J Med Pharmac Sci 1988;20:947–956.
7. Takahashi H et al. Blood and Vessel 1989;20:240–249.
8. Okabe K, Kato I et al. Gastroenterogia Jpn 1992;27:61–68.
9. Nakamura T, Nishizawa T et al. Nature 1989;342–440.
10. Noji S, Tashiro K et al. Biochem Biophys Res Commun 1990;173:42–47.
11. Wolf HK, Zarnegar R et al. Hepatology 1991;14:488–494.
12. Jezequel AM, Mancini R. Hepatology 1987;5:174–178.
13. Higashio K, Shima N et al. Biochem Biophys Res Commun 1990;170:1151–1158.
14. Shima N, Tsuda E et al. Biochem Biophys Res Commun 1994;200:808–815.
15. Armendariz-Borunda J, Seyer IM et al. FASEB J 1990;4:215–221.
16. Nagy P, Schaff Z et al. Hepatology 1991;14:269–273.
17. Michael SP, Matsumoto K et al. J Biol Chem 1992;267:20493–20496.
18. Wojta J, Nkamura T et al. Blood 1994;84:151–157.
19. Morimoto A, Tada K et al. Jpn J Cancer Res 1994;85:53–62.
20. Santos OFP, Nigam SK. Dev Biol 1993;160:293–302.
21. Falcone DJ, McCaffrey TA et al. J Biol Chem 1993;268:11951–11958.
22. Rieder H, Armbrust T et al. Hepatology 1993;18:937–944.
23. Francavilla A, Starzl TE et al. Hepatology 1991;14:665–670.
24. Fujiwara K, Nagoshi S et al. Hepatology 1993;18:1443–1449.
25. Ishiki Y, Ohnishi H et al. Hepatology 1991; 16:1227–1235.
26. Nakayama Y, Kohno K et al. Cancer J 1993;6:213–219.
27. Koj A, Korzus E, Baumann H et al. Biol Chem Hoppe-Seyler 1993;374:193–201.

Progress in Hepatology Vol. 1.
Cellular and Molecular Biology.
M. Yamanaka, K. Okabe and G. Toda, editors.

Mechanism of liver cell injury induced by hepatitis C virus

Norio Hayashi, Tetsuo Takehara, Eiji Mita, Naoki Hiramatsu, Akinori Kasahara, Hideyuki Fusamoto and Takenobu Kamada
First Department of Medicine, Osaka University School of Medicine, Osaka, Japan

Abstract. To investigate the mechanism of liver cell injury in type C hepatitis, we examined the correlation between liver cell damage and the expression of Fas antigen and found more expression of Fas antigen in liver tissue with active inflammation. Also, we isolated a cDNA clone for human Fas ligand and confirmed the expression of Fas ligand in liver-infiltrating mononuclear cells obtained from patients with chronic hepatitis C. These findings suggest that Fas ligand–Fas antigen system may play an important role in liver cell injury by hepatitis C virus (HCV) infection.

The lack of a small animal model of HCV infection has impeded elucidation of the pathogenesis of this virus. We developed an HCV-expressing animal model using cationic liposome-mediated in vivo gene transfer. The full length of the HCV genome was successfully expressed in adult rat liver using this procedure. Also, immunohistochemical analysis revealed the HCV core protein in a small number of hepatocytes scattered in the lobules.

Key words: apoptosis, Fas ligand, gene delivery, type C hepatitis.

Introduction

The isolation of hepatitis C virus (HCV) genome by Chiron has greatly advanced the characterization of the main agents which cause viral hepatitis in humans [1,2]. The HCV genome is a positive-stranded RNA molecule of approximately 10 kilobases and codes for a polyprotein [3]. The 5′-terminal sequence is thought to be the structural region coding for core and envelope proteins with the larger remaining part coding for nonstructural proteins. Although the HCV genome has been cloned, little is known about the mechanism of the hepatocellular injury induced by HCV. So, we examined the mechanism of liver cell injury induced by HCV infection.

HCV genotype and RNA titer in type C chronic liver disease

Various complete HCV-cDNA clones have been isolated since the HCV prototype was discovered. From homologies of nucleotide sequences, the

Address for correspondence: Norio Hayashi, M.D., First Department of Medicine, Osaka University School of Medicine, Yamadaoka 2-2, Suita-shi, Osaka 565, Japan

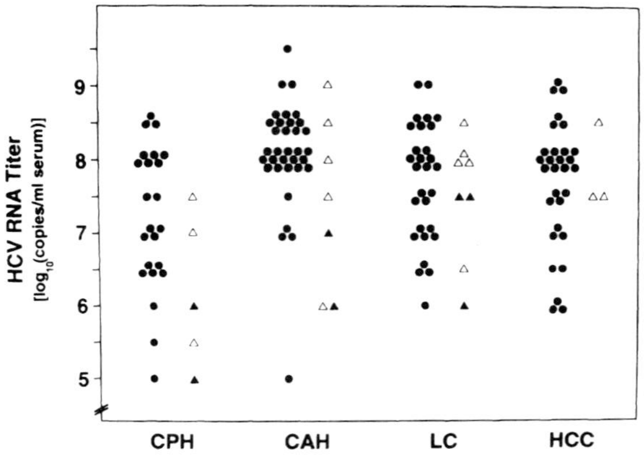

Fig. 1. Correlation between HCV genotype and RNA titer in various categories of type C chronic liver disease. ●, type Ib; △, type IIa; ▲, type IIb.

clones were classified into several genotypes. We classified HCV into four genotypes by using genotype-specific PCR primers in the core region [4,5]. Type Ia was observed in 105 cases (77%), whereas types IIa and IIb were found in 16 (11%) and 9 (6%), respectively. Type Ia was observed in only 1 patient, and double infection was found in 4 patients. Thus, type Ib was the most common genotype among Japanese patients.

Type C hepatitis follows a slow sequential progression from chronic hepatitis through liver cirrhosis to hepatocellular carcinoma (HCC). We examined the correlation between HCV genotype and HVC-RNA titer in various stages of type C chronic liver disease (Fig. 1). We quantified the amount of HCV-RNA in serum by a competitive RT-PCR assay [6,7]. There was no significant difference in the prevalence of HCV genotype in each stage of chronic liver disease. We also found the HCV-RNA titer to be significantly higher in chronic active hepatitis (CAH) than in chronic persistent hepatitis (CPH). This significant difference was also observed for type Ib patients. When the titers were compared between types IIa and IIb, there was no significant difference at any stage of type C chronic liver disease [8].

The expression of Fas antigen in liver

Furthermore, to examine the distribution of HCV-RNA-positive cells in the liver, we detected HCV-RNA by in situ hybridization technique using synthetic DNA probes derived from the 5′-untranslated and core regions of HCV genome [9]. Three DNA probes consisting of 40 nucleotides each were synthesized, and labeled in the 3′ end with (^{35}S)dATP. Clusters of silver grains indicating hybridization with HCV-RNA were observed mainly over the cytoplasm of hepatocytes. Next, we examined the relationship between HCV-related antigen expression and the histological characteristics. The mean ALT levels in the HCV-positive group tended to be higher than those in the HCV-negative group. On comparison between HCV-related antigen expression and liver histological appearance with HAI scoring system, no significant differences in portal inflammation and fibrosis were observed, but periportal necrosis and intralobular inflammation were found to be more severe in the positive samples than in the negative ones [10].

The mechanism of liver injury with type C hepatitis remains to be clarified. It is now generally accepted that cytotoxic T lymphocytes (CTL) are involved in the immune clearance of HCV-infected hepatocytes and in the pathogenesis of HCV infection. The incomplete immune clearance is considered to cause the chronicity of HCV infection. Hagi et al. demonstrated that perforin- and Fas-based mechanisms account for all T cell-mediated cytotoxicity [11]. Thus, the Fas ligand–Fas antigen system is thought to contribute to liver cell injury by HCV infection. Recently, Itoh et al. cloned cDNA for the human Fas antigen [12,13], which is a cell surface protein that mediates apoptosis with treatment of the antibody to Fas antigen in vivo, and cells with Fas antigen expression seem to be led to death by apoptosis. Molecular cloning reveals that the Fas antigen belongs to the receptor family that includes TNF receptor, nerve growth factor and CD40 antigen

Apoptosis has been also shown to be the type of cell death occurring in acute and chronic hepatitis, where the apoptotic bodies have traditionally been referred to as acidophilic or Councilman bodies [13]. However, the role of apoptosis in type C hepatitis has not been studied adequately, because apoptotic bodies are histologically visible for only a few hours. Then, we examined immunohistochemically the expression of Fas antigen in type C hepatitis [14]. Expression of Fas antigen was found mainly in the cytoplasm of hepatocytes and these positive cells were found especially among infiltrating lymphocytes.

We examined the prevalence of Fas antigen expression in type C chronic hepatitis. In the patients with CAH, 83% of the samples were positive, while only 38% of samples were positive in the patients with CPH. High prevalence of Fas antigen expression was shown in liver tissue with more severe inflammation. For further study, we examined the relationship between the expression of Fas antigen and histological appearance scored by HAI scoring system. The inflammation in both periportal and portal areas was found to be more severe in the samples of the Fas antigen-positive group than in those of the Fas antigen-negative group. Next, we examined the relationship between Fas antigen expression and HCV core antigen expression. The prevalence of Fas antigen expression in the HCV antigen-positive group (92%) was higher than that in the HCV antigen-negative group (58%). These findings suggest that Fas antigen expression plays an important role in the active inflammation of type C hepatitis.

Fas Ag expression, however, does not mean apoptosis by itself. The cell with Fas Ag expression is a candidate for apoptosis. To detect the apoptotic cell directly, the TdT-mediated dUTP-biotin nick and labeling method (TUNEL method) was used. This method is: after protease treatment, biotinylated nucleotides are in situ incorporated into DNA breaks in apoptotic cells and subsequently stained with DAB via peroxidase-conjugated avidin. Positive stainings were found in the nuclei of the hepatocytes, and we were able to detect the DNA fragmentation in the liver tissue of the patients with chronic hepatitis C.

The expression of Fas ligand in liver-infiltrating mononuclear cells

These observations strongly suggest that Fas system-induced apoptosis plays an important role in liver cell injury by HCV infection. However, little information was obtained about the Fas ligand. Suda et al. isolated rat Fas ligand cDNA. We also isolated a cDNA clone for human Fas ligand to examine the role of Fas ligand in the apoptosis of hepatocytes induced by HCV infection [15]. Approximately 1.9 kb of human Fas ligand cDNA was clarified. The open reading-frame encodes 281 amino acids. The amino acids sequence of human Fas ligand indicates 76% and 77% identity with those of rat and mouse ligand, respectively. The N-terminal portion of 79 amino acids contains 32 residues of proline and is considered to be the putative cytoplasmic domain. The putative transmembrane domain shows much hydrophobicity. The extracellular domain, 179 C-terminal amino acids, is considered to interact with Fas antigen and its amino acid sequence has 78% and 81% identity with those of rat and mouse Fas ligand extracellular domains, respectively.

Next, we examined the expression of Fas ligand in liver-infiltrating mononuclear cells obtained from patients with chronic hepatitis C. The amplified products (231 bp) derived from Fas ligand transcripts were detected in liver-infiltrating mononuclear cells. However, no signal was detected in liver tissues (Fig. 2). These findings suggest that the Fas ligand–Fas antigen system may play an important role in liver cell injury by HCV infection (Fig. 3).

In vivo transfection of HCV cDNA to rat liver with cationic liposome-mediated gene delivery

The lack of a small animal model of HCV has impeded elucidation of the pathogenesis of this virus. The ability to express the HCV genome in a small

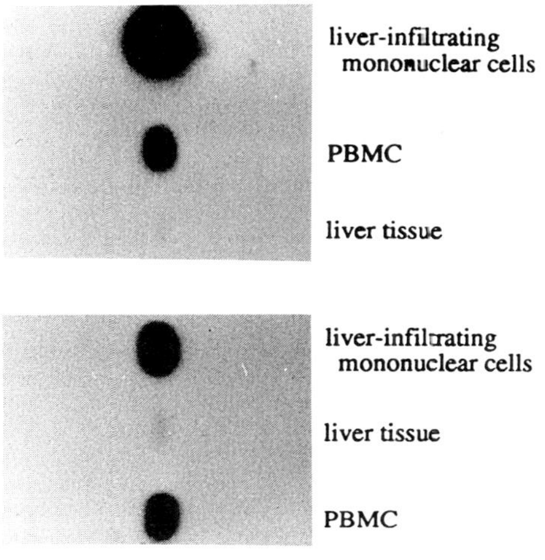

Fig. 2. Detection of Fas ligand transcripts in liver-infiltrating mononuclear cells and liver tissue.

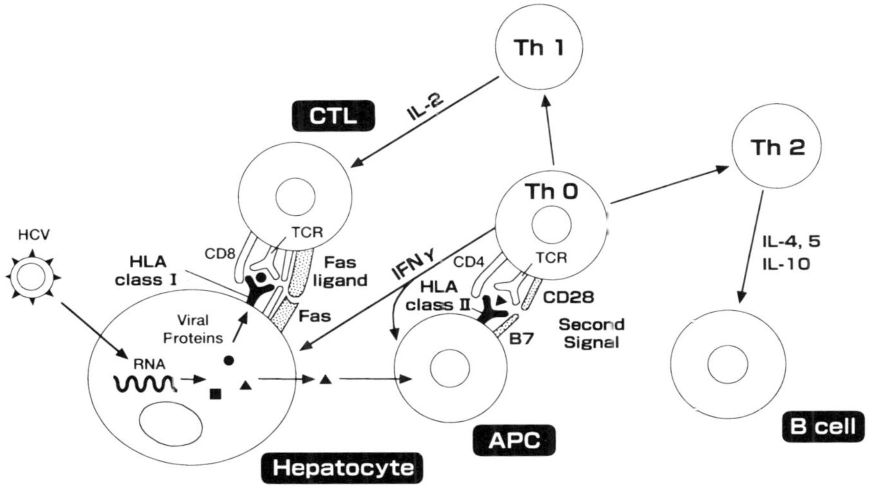

Fig. 3. Schematic representation of the molecular mechanism of liver cell injury induced by HCV infection.

animal would create new opportunities for elucidating the pathophysiological roles of this virus. A number of methods have been developed for in vivo gene expression in the liver. These include encapsulation of DNA in various forms of liposomes [16,17], delivery of DNA complexed with specific protein carriers [18,19], and infection using viral vectors [20,21]. However, the transfection efficiency of the liposome-mediated procedure varies with different reports and liposome formulations. The uptake of DNA through receptor-mediated gene delivery is quantitatively limited by the fact that most of the administered DNA is degraded in the endosomes during the gene transfer process. Virus-mediated procedures are efficient but recombinant viral particles are cumbersome to prepare. Thus, a simple DNA carrier system for hepatocytes in vivo should be developed.

Cationic liposomes containing N[1-(2,3-dioleyloxy)propyl]-N,N,N-triethylammonium (DOTMA), which is called lipofectin, have been used to deliver DNA into cultured cells [22,23]. Cationic liposomes that are 250 nm in diameter spontaneously interact with negatively charged DNA. The resultant cationic liposomes-coated DNA has a net positive charge and thus can associate with the negatively charged surface of cells. This procedure is different from the traditional liposome-mediated procedure because DNA is not encapsulated in the liposomes. Recently, cationic liposomes were shown to be useful as an in vivo DNA carrier system for arterial wall [24,25], brain [26,27], and airway epithelial cells [28,29]. This procedure could provide researchers with a rapid and reproducible source of animals with which to elucidate the functions of genes transferred and expressed in vivo. However, there has been no attempt to use such cationic liposomes to introduce foreign genes into liver cells. Then, we introduced the full length of the HCV genome into rat liver to develop an animal model of HCV infection using this procedure [30].

Male Sprague-Dawley rats weighing 200 g were anesthetized with pentobarbital and then their viscera were exposed through a midline incision. The common bile duct was identified and cannulated with a 27-gauge needle; 1.0 ml of DNA liposome complexes was injected retrogradely into the biliary tract. The common bile duct was ligated for 90 minutes to keep the DNA lipsome complexes in the liver. The ligature was then removed. Finally, the abdominal incision was closed and the animals were allowed to recover.

pActLacZ contains the *Escherichia coli* LacZ gene preceded by the chicken β-actin promoter. The presence of β-galactosidase-expressing cells in liver transfected with pActLacZ was clearly detected as deep blue cells in X-Gal-stained cryostat sections. The specificity of the X-Gal histochemical reaction was demonstrated by analysis of pAGS3M091-transfected liver, which contained no blue-stained cells. β-Galactosidase-expressing cells were scattered in the liver lobules and were morphologically hepatocytes (Fig. 4). Although a few hepatocytes next to the portal area were stained blue, no positive cells were observed in the portal tract.

To determine the optimal ratio of DNA to lipofectin, liver tissues were evaluated for LacZ expression 2 days after transfection. At least 15 sections were obtained from each rat liver. The transfection efficiency was expressed as the average number of blue β-galactosidase-expressing cells in 50 mm^2 of a liver section. Figure 5 shows the effect of varying the total amount of DNA added while keeping the amount of lipofectin constant at 200 or 100 μg. The

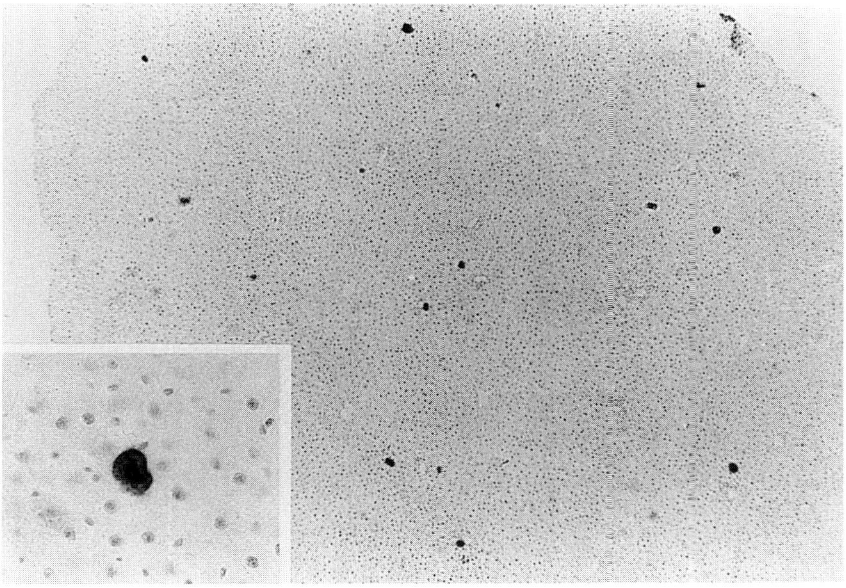

Fig. 4. X-Gal histochemical staining of rat liver transfected with pActLacZ. The rat was sacrificed 2 days after receiving pActLacZ complexed with lipofectin. β-Galactosidase-expressing cells are scattered in the liver lobules. Main panel ×40, inset ×400.

mass ratio of DNA:lipofectin of 1:4 gave maximal β-galactosidase expression. Based on this observation, 50 μg of the vector DNA complexed with 200 μg of lipofectin was used for subsequent studies. The time-course of LacZ gene expression following tranfection was examined. Expression of β-galactosidase was observed as early as 1 day after transfection but had decreased by day 7 (Fig. 6). So, in vivo gene delivery of this system resulted in transient gene expression.

In this in vivo gene transfer, foreign gene expression was observed only in hepatocytes, but not in the biliary epithelium. In in vitro experiments, lipofectin was shown to be useful for transferring DNA into rat primary hepatocytes [31–33]. It may be possible that lipofectin more efficiently transfects hepatocytes than biliary epithelial cells. In a study on relative promoter strength in rat primary hepatocytes, β-actin promoters as well as cytomegalovirus and SRα promoters found to exhibit strong transcriptional activity [32]. There may be a difference in the strength of the β-actin promoter between hepatocytes and the biliary epithelium. However, the mechanism responsible for selective gene expression in hepatocytes is unknown.

The full-length sequence of HCV cDNA (M094) was isolated from the serum of a Japanese chronic hepatitis C patient. This clone contains 9,426 bp,

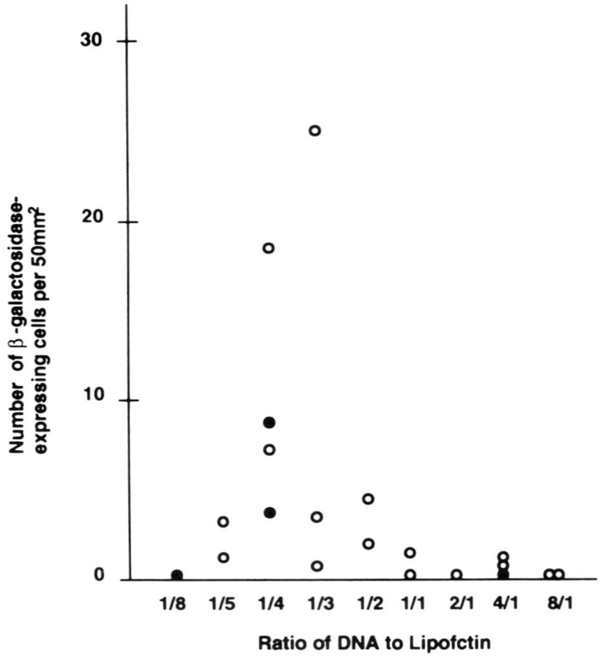

Fig. 5. The effect of the DNA to lipofectin ratio on β-galactosidase expression in vivo. Shown are data for rats two days after the administration of various amounts of pActLacZ, the amount of lipofectin being kept constant at 200 μg (○) or 100 μg (●).

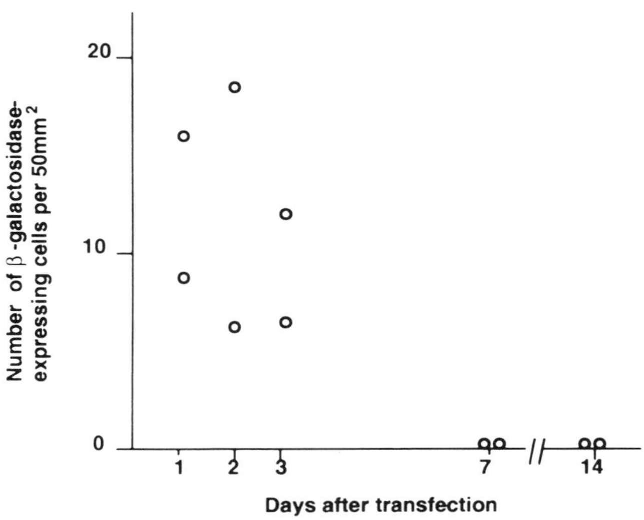

Fig. 6. Time-course of β-galactosidase expression in rat liver transfected with pActLacZ and lipofectin.

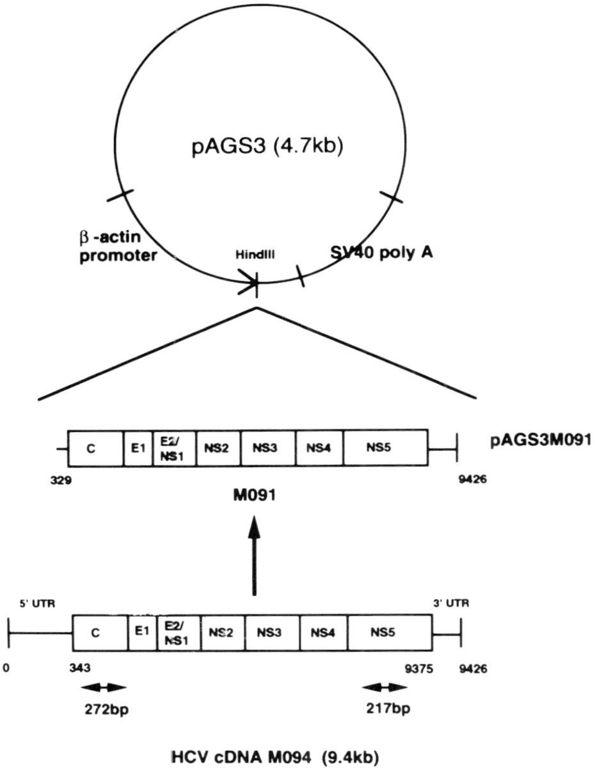

Fig. 7. Schematic representation of expression vector pAGS3M091. M094 is the full-length HCV cDNA which contains a 9,033 bp protein coding sequence (box), and 342 and 51 bp 5′ and 3′ UTR (bars). The numbers represent the nucleotide positions of M094. M091 was generated from M094 such that nucleotides 329 to 9,426 were present and then inserted into the Hind III site just after chicken β-actin promoter of pAGS3 to create pAGS3M091. Double arrows indicate the positions of DNA fragments after PCR amplification.

which is 10 nucleotides longer than the previously published sequence [34], and encodes a 3,010-amino acid polyprotein. In addition, there are 342 and 51 base 5′ and 3′ untranslated regions (UTR), respectively. M091 was generated from M094 such that nucleotides 329 to 9,426 were present. M091 was inserted into the Hind III site just after chicken β-actin promoter of pAGS3 (32) to create pAGS3M091 (Fig. 7).

Two days following retrograde biliary injection of pAGS3M091, the presence of HCV transcripts was confirmed in rat liver by RNA PCR analysis (Fig. 8). To ensure that only RNA sequences were being detected, each sample was evaluated in the absence or presence of reverse transcriptase. Using two sets of primer pairs designed for the core and NS5 regions, HCV transcripts were detected in pAGS3M091-transfected liver (lanes 2 and 4).

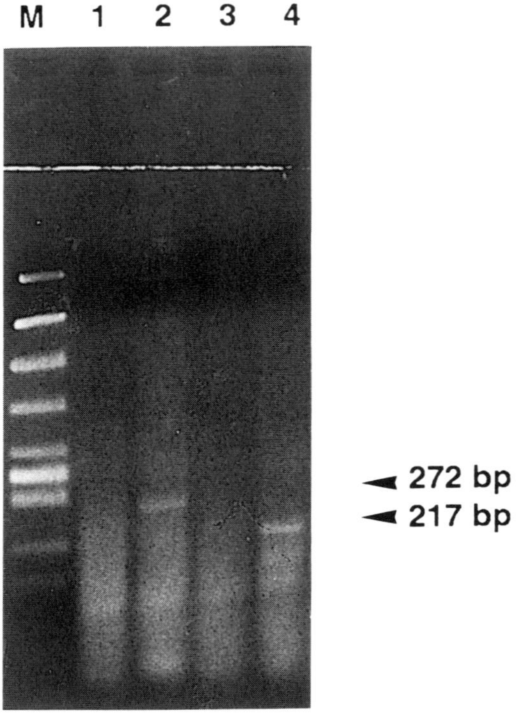

Fig. 8. Specific RT/PCR amplification of the core (lanes 1 and 2) and NS5 (lanes 3 and 4) regions of the HCV transcripts from pAGS3M091-injected rat liver. M, molecular mass markers: Hind II-digested ox174. PCR was performed with (lanes 2 and 4) or without (lanes 1 and 3) an RT step. The expected 272 and 217 bp fragments for the core and NS5 regions, respectively, were amplified from the pAGS3M091-injected rat liver.

These signals did not arise from contaminating HCV cDNA, since none of the samples showed specific amplification in the absence of reverse transcriptase (lanes 1 and 3). These results showed that the 5′ and 3′ portions of the pAGS3M091-directed HCV transcript were present in the liver transfected with pAGS3M091.

Two days after pAGS3M091 transfection, expression of the HCV core protein was analyzed by immunohistochemistry. A few hepatocytes containing immunoreactive protein were scattered in the lobules (Fig. 9). Immunostaining of the HCV core protein was observed in the cytoplasm of hepatocytes in a granular fashion. No positive immunostaining was observed in pAGS3M091-transfected rat liver when a purified IgG was used instead of the anti-HCV core antibody. The specificity of the immunohistochemical analysis was also confirmed in control pActLacZ-transfected rats, the HCV core protein not being found. The expression of HCV genome was transient, since

A

B

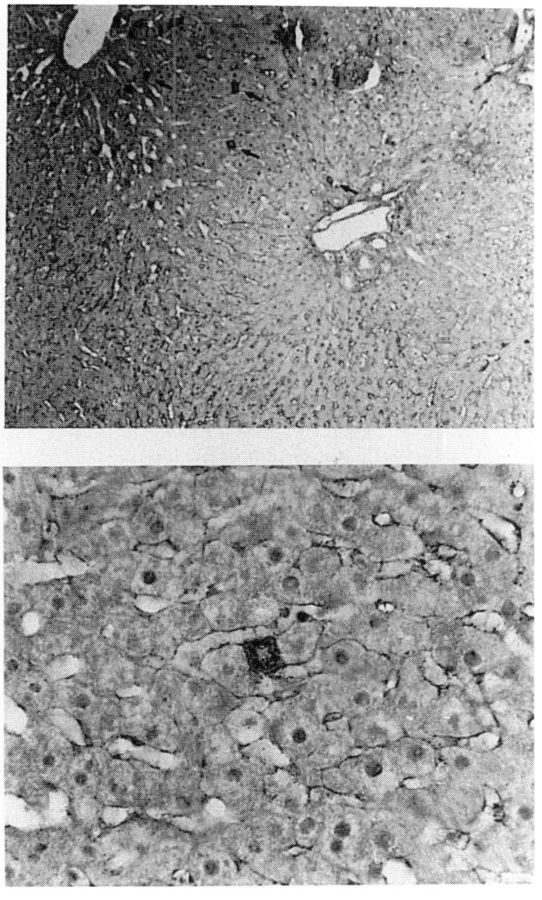

Fig. 9. Immunohistochemical staining of the HCV core protein. A: Hepatocytes exhibiting positive staining are scattered in the lobules. ×100. B: Each positive hepatocyte is strongly stained in the cytoplasm. ×400.

both the HCV transcripts and the HCV core proteins were not observed 7 days after transfection.

Using the cationic liposome-mediated procedure, the HCV genome was successfully expressed in adult rat liver. This was confirmed by the presence of HCV transcripts and the HCV core protein in the transfected liver. We previously demonstrated that the number of HCV-infected hepatocytes was small in chronic hepatitis C patients by an in situ hybridization technique [9] and an immunohistochemical study [10]. In this HCV-expressing animal, a small number of HCV core-positive hepatocytes was found scattered in the lobules, resembling human HCV infection. Although HCV expression is transient in this system, multiple injection of DNA by way of cannulation of the bile duct would provide us long-term HCV expression. This model will be useful for examining the immunopathological role of HCV in vivo.

References

1. Yuki N, Hayashi N, Hagiwara H et al. Dig Dis Sci 1992;37:1483–1488.
2. Hagiwara H, Hayashi, N, Mita E et al. Gastroenterology 1993;102:692–694.
3. Choo QL, Kuo G, Weiner AJ et al. Science 1989;244:359–362.
4. Okamoto H, Sugiyama Y, Okada S et al. J Gen Virol 1993;73:673–679.
5. Mita E, Hayashi N, Kanazawa Y et al. Dig Dis Sci 1994;39:977–982.
6. Hagiwara H, Hayashi N, Mita E et al. Gastroenterology 1993;104:877–883.
7. Hagiwara H, Hayashi N, Mita E et al. Hepatology 1993;17:545–550.
8. Mita E, Hayashi N, Kanazawa Y et al. J Hepatol 1994;21:468–473.
9. Haruna Y, Hayashi N, Hiramatsu N et al. J Hepatol 1993;18:96–100.
10. Hiramatsu N, Hayashi N, Haruna Y et al. Hepatology 1993;16:306–311.
11. Kagi D, Vignaux F, Ledermann B et al. Science 1994;265:528–530.
12. Itoh N, Yonehara S, Ishii A et al. Cell 1993;66:233–243.
13. Kerr JFR, Cooksley WGE, Searle J et al. Lancet 1979;2:827–828.
14. Hiramatsu N, Hayashi N, Katayama K et al. Hepatology 1994;19:1360–1365.
15. Mita E, Hayashi N, Iio S et al. Biochem Biophys Res Commun 1994;204:468–474.
16. Kaneda Y, Iwai K, Uchida T. Science 1989;243:375–378.
17. Kato K, Nakanishi M, Kaneda Y et al. J Biol Chem 1991;266:3361–3364.
18. Wu GY, Wu CH. J Biol Chem 1988;263:14621–14624.
19. Wu GY, Wilson JM, Shalaby F et al. J Biol Chem 1991;266:14338–14342.
20. Jaffe HA, Danel C, Longenecker G et al. Nature Genet 1992;1:372–378.
21. Morsy MA, Alford EL, Bett A et al. J Clin Invest 1993;92:1580–1586.
22. Felgner PL, Gadek TR, Holm M et al. Proc Natl Acad Sci USA 1987;84:7413–7417.
23. Felgner PL, Ringold GM. Nature 1989;337:387–388.
24. Nabel EG, Plautz G, Nabel GJ. Science 1990;249:1285–1288.
25. Nabel EG, Yang Z, Plautz G et al. Nature 1993;362:844–846.
26. Holt CE, Garlick N, Cornel E. Neuron 1990;4:203–214.
27. Ono T, Fujino Y, Tsuchiya T et al. Neurosci Lett 1990;117:259–263.
28. Yoshimura K, Rosenfeld MA, Nakamura H et al. Nucleic Acids Res 1992;20:3233–3240.
29. Hyde SC, Gill DR, Higgins CF et al. Nature 1993;362:250–255.
30. Takehara T, Hayashi N, Miyamoto Y et al. Expression of the hepatitis C virus genome in rat liver after cationic liposome-mediated in vivo gene transfer. Hepatology, (in press).
31. Jacoby DB, Zilz ND, Towle HC. J Biol Chem 1989;264:17623–17626.
32. Ponder KP, Dunbar RP, Wilson DR et al. Hum Gene Ther 1991;2:41–52.
33. Jarnagin WR, Debs RJ, Wang SS et al. Nucleic Acids Res 1992;20:4205–4211.
34. Takamizawa A, Mori C, Fuke I et al. J Virol 1991;65:1105–1113.

Progress in Hepatology Vol. 1.
Cellular and Molecular Biology.
M. Yamanaka, K. Okabe and G. Toda, editors.

Molecular mechanisms of persistent infection and interferon resistance of hepatitis C virus

Nobuyuki Enomoto,[1] Masayuki Kurosaki[1] and Chifumi Sato[2]
[1]Second Department of Internal Medicine and [2]Division of Health Science, Faculty of Medicine, Tokyo Medical and Dental University, Bunkyo-ku, Tokyo 113, Japan

Abstract. The hypervariable region of predominant hepatitis C virus (HCV) genomes detected in serum by direct sequencing changes rapidly and serially along the course of acute and chronic HCV infection, suggesting that these changes in the hypervariable region may be one of the mechanisms of recurrence and persistence of HCV infection. These changes are also observed during interferon treatment. Analysis of populations of circulating HCV genomes by the single strand conformation polymorphism (SSCP) method targeted to the hypervariable region has further clarified that they are composed of quasispecies and that predominant HCV quasispecies change during chronic infection and interferon treatment. These changes appear to result from either evolution or selection of the hypervariable region in vivo. Similar changes in the liver are also suggested. There are interferon-sensitive and interferon-resistant quasispecies, and this difference in the sensitivity may be determined by the specific sequence of a part of the NS5 region.

Key words: hypervariable region, quasispecies, single strand conformation polymorphism.

Introduction

In most cases, hepatitis C virus (HCV) infection is followed by persistent or recurrent relapses resulting in liver cirrhosis and hepatocellular carcinoma (HCC). Mechanisms of persistent infection, however, have not yet been understood. Genomic characterizations have shown that there is a hypervariable region (HVR) in the upstream end of the E2/NS1 gene of HCV genomes [1,2]. The HVR has been shown to exhibit marked sequence variations among different HCV isolates [3,4]. Ogata et al. [5] have reported that even in a single patient, 28.2% of the nucleotides in the HVR are substituted in 13 years. Weiner et al. [6] have suggested that there are epitopes recognized by B cells in the HVR and that the HCV appearing after relapses has different HVR from that of the earlier phase. Antibodies directed to the previous HVR are produced while those directed to the latter are not present. The E2/NS1 region of the HCV genome corresponds to the second envelope glycoprotein

Address for correspondence: Nobuyuki Enomoto, M.D., Second Department of Internal Medicine, Faculty of Medicine, Tokyo Medical and Dental University, 1-5-45 Yushima, Bunkyo-ku, Tokyo 113, Japan.

of the pestivirus that contains epitopes for neutralizing antibodies and is involved in protective immunity [7]. In human immunodeficiency virus (HIV), significant variations of viral envelope proteins have also been demonstrated; the gp120 V3 domain of HIV genomes contains major epitopes for neutralizing antibodies, and escape mutants evolve as a result of continuous immune selection [8,9].

To study mechanisms of persistent infection of HCV, we analyzed sequential changes in the HVR during acute and chronic infection, and also during interferon (IFN) treatment by direct sequencing.

Analysis of sequential changes in the HVR by direct sequencing

Analytical methods

RNA was extracted from plasma samples by the acid guanidinium thiocyanate-phenol-chloroform method [10] with slight modifications. cDNA was synthesized in 5 ml of the reverse transcription (RT) mixture adjusted to contain 1 ml of the RNA solution, 50 units of Moloney murine leukemia virus reverse transcriptase (Bethesda Research Laboratories Life Technologies Inc., Gaithersburg, USA), 10 units of RNase inhibitor (Promega, Madison, USA), 50 pg of random hexamer (Takara, Kyoto, Japan), 50 mM Tris-HCl (pH 8.3), 75 mM KCl, 3 mM $MgCl_2$ and 10 mM dithiothreitol. The mixture was incubated at 37°C for 45 min.

Five millilitres of the cDNA solution was made up to 25 ml of a PCR mixture containing 10 mM Tris-HCl (pH 8.3), 50 mM KCl, 1.5 mM $MgCl_2$, 10 pmol of each PCR primer, 200 mM each dNTP, 0.01% gelatin and 0.5 units of Taq polymerase (Perkin Elmer Cetus, Norwalk, USA) [11]. For the amplification of HCV cDNA containing the HVR, PCR consisting of 50 cycles of denaturing at 94°C for 1 min, annealing at 60°C for 1 min, and polymerization at 72°C for 1 min was performed. Amplified HCV cDNA fragments were purified by the electrophoresis with low melting point agarose gel. Single stranded cDNA was amplified by the asymmetric PCR with the purified cDNA as a template. Residual dNTPs and primers were removed using the spin filtration column (Suprec-02, Takara, Kyoto, Japan).

The nucleotide sequences were determined by the dideoxy chain termination method using the modified T7 DNA polymerase (Sequenase version 2.0 kit, United States Biochemical, Cleveland, OH, USA).

Sequential variations in acute infection

RNA was extracted from plasma samples of two patients with sporadic hepatitis and one with posttransfusion hepatitis. cDNA containing the HVR was amplified by the RT-PCR method and was directly sequenced to determine predominant sequences [12].

A 33-year-old female presented herself to the hospital for elevated serum transferases; the prolonged elevation gradually resolved over 28 weeks. HCV-RNA disappeared once at 12 weeks after the onset, and then reappeared at 52 weeks. There were no alterations of deduced amino acid sequences in the HVR at the time of exacerbation at 9 weeks from the onset. The HCV obtained 52 weeks later had seven amino acid substitutions compared with that obtained in the initial phase.

A 57-year-old female was transfused several packs of fresh frozen plasma for the treatment of fulminant hepatitis A. Serum transferase levels elevated 18 weeks after the transfusion, and the abnormalities in serum transferases continued thereafter. Serum anti-C100 became positive at the time of the exacerbation. Plasma HCV-RNA was detected 18 and 57 weeks after the transfusion. Comparison of the sequences revealed a marked diversity in the HVR with the homology of 30% that was not significantly different from the published sequence of HCV-J4 (52%).

A 41-year-old female developed acute sporadic non-A, non-B hepatitis. Initial elevation of serum transferases returned to normal in six weeks. Plasma HCV-RNA was detectable one week after the clinical onset and persisted for two weeks, whereas anti-C100 remained negative during the acute phase. Her serum transferase levels continued to be normal until 55 weeks after the first onset, then serum transferase levels elevated again concomitantly with anti-C100 seroconversion and the recurrence of viremia. A liver biopsy showed chronic active hepatitis. The HCV of the recurrent phase had one amino acid substitution of tyrosine by histidine at residue 394 in the HVR compared with that of the initial phase. In the chronic phase, HCV also had the same substitution and three additional amino acid changes in the HVR. Zero to 34 nucleotide changes were present in the HVR during the course of acute hepatitis C. Of the nucleotide changes, 88–100% were associated with amino acid alterations.

Thus, we have shown that the HVR of HCV genome changes rapidly and serially along the course of acute HCV infection for the first time, suggesting that the evolution of the HVR may be one of the mechanisms of recurrence and persistence of HCV infection. It is, however, necessary to study whether these changes are also observed in patients with chronic hepatitis.

Sequential variations in chronic infection

To further evaluate the significance of sequence variations in the HVR of HCV during chronic infection, pairwise comparison of predominant nucleotide sequences separately obtained was performed in patients with chronic hepatitis C [13]. HCV-RNA was extracted from paired plasma samples obtained from patients with chronic hepatitis C over an approximately one-year interval. cDNA containing the HVR was amplified by the RT-PCR method and was directly sequenced to determine predominant sequences.

Predominant sequences of the HVR at the second time point were different from those at the first time point in all the individuals, and significant sequence variations were observed during this relatively short period. Of these nucleotide substitutions, 90% were shown to result in changes of predicted amino acid sequences. These findings suggested that antigenicity of the epitopes composed of these amino acids changed during these periods, and the selection of these variants occurred in vivo. There were differences in the rate of nucleotide sequence variations of the HVR between four patients with episodes of the flare-up of ALT levels ($1.54–2.24 \times 10^{-1}$ per genome site per year) and eight patients with the quiescent course ($0.13–1.21 \times 10^{-1}$ per genome site per year).

These findings demonstrate that the rapid sequence variations of the HVR of predominant virus takes place during the natural course of chronic HCV infection. These sequence variations seem to occur as adaptive responses of HCV to escape from the host immunosurveillance system and may play a major role in persistent infection as well as in the occasional flare-up of hepatitis activity. Therefore, it is also interesting to study how IFN treatment affects these sequential variations of the HVR.

Sequential variations during IFN treatment

Weiner et al. reported a patient whose relapse after interferon therapy was associated with an appearance of an escape variant in the HVR [6]. More recently, Okada et al. reported three nonresponders to interferon treatment, whose HVR population underwent significant changes [14]. The rate of mutation may not be equivalent with untreated patients, because interferon therapy may have accelerated the mutation of the HVR in their cases. To investigate the effect of IFN treatment on the mutation rate, and the role of HVR variants in the mechanism of IFN resistance, HVR sequences were compared before and after recombinant IFN-α-2b treatment. cDNA containing the HVR was obtained from serial plasma samples of each patient and directly sequenced to determine the changes in the predominant sequence [15].

In some patients, HCV-RNA was eliminated by IFN treatment. In the other patients, HCV-RNA was not eradicated. The predominant HCV which remained after IFN treatment was mutant HCV with nucleotide changes in the HVR resulting in amino acid substitutions. The majority of the nucleotide substitutions was nonsynonymous, indicating positive selections for mutants with amino acid changes in the HVR. The mutation rate was significantly higher in patients whose plasma HCV-RNA was continuously detected during and after IFN treatment than in patients whose plasma HCV-RNA became undetectable during the treatment and reappeared after the cessation of the treatment, suggesting that the evolution of the HVR in each patient seemed to be associated with the effect of IFN treatment. Thus, HVR variants play an important role in maintaining persistent infection under IFN treatment by evading the host immunosurveillance system.

Analysis of sequential variations of the HVR of HCV by the single strand conformation polymorphism

HVR variants play an important role in maintaining persistent infection in acute and chronic infection and during IFN treatment by evading the host immunosurveillance system. Previous studies on HCV heterogeneity were mainly performed by cloning of PCR products [2,14] or by direct sequencing of PCR products [12,15]. Direct sequencing is a simple method to detect major sequences. The HCV population in vivo, however, consists of heterogeneous mixtures of genetically different but closely related variants defined as a "quasispecies" [16,17] and minor clones could be overlooked by direct sequencing. On the other hand, the cloning-sequencing method could not reveal the composition of whole HCV quasispecies populations, since there are millions of HCV clones in serum and selection of 10 or 20 clones could not represent the whole population.

Single strand conformation polymorphism (SSCP) analysis [18] is a method that detects sequence differences of single stranded DNA by non denaturing polyacrylamide gel electrophoresis (PAGE). Partially denatured DNA in the gel takes sequence-specific three-dimensional conformation, and even a single nucleotide difference can be detected as a mobility shift. Therefore, complex mixtures of DNA species can be separated into bands with different mobility even if they are the same size. However, there are no reports that applied the SSCP method to the analysis of viral genomes except one brief report [19], in which SSCP profiles were utilized to evaluate the sequence heterogeneity among hepatitis B virus isolates. We then applied the SSCP method to HCV genome analysis to evaluate serial changes in its quasispecies populations within isolates and to clarify the role of HCV quasispecies in persistent infection and IFN resistance [20].

Analytical methods

Serum HCV-RNA was extracted and converted to cDNA as described above. Five microlitres of the cDNA solution was made up to 25 μl of a PCR mixture containing 10 nM Tris-HCl (pH 8.3), 50 mM KCl, 1.5 mM $MgCl_2$, 400 mM of each PCR primer (outer primer), 200 μM each dNTP, 0.01% gelatin and 0.5 units of Taq polymerase (AmpliTaq, Cetus Corp., Emeryville, CA, USA) [11]. For the amplification of HCV cDNA containing the HVR, PCR consisting of 50 cycles of denaturing at 94°C for 1 min, annealing at 60°C for

1 min, and polymerization at 72°C for 1 min was performed. Single stranded cDNA was amplified by the nested asymmetric PCR with one hundredth of the first PCR product as a template. Either 5′- or 3′-nested (inner) primer was reduced to 40 nM in the nested asymmetric PCR.

Five microlitres of the nested PCR product was mixed with 10 μl of a SSCP loading solution (0.05% xylene cyanol, 20 mM EDTA and 95% formamide) and was subjected to modified nondenatured PAGE in 0.6X TBE buffer with 100 V for 6 h. The gel was made of 0.5X MDE gel (Hoefer, San Francisco, CA, USA). The gel was stained with ethidium bromide, and the bands were detected and photographed on the ultraviolet transilluminator. The same experiments were performed using end-labeled nested primers. Nonlimiting nested primers were end-labeled with [g-^{32}P]ATP using T4 polynucleotide kinase. The SSCP gel was vacuum-dried and exposed to X-ray films (isotopic-SSCP).

Separated bands were excised from the SSCP gel under the ultraviolet light. Pieces of the gel were crushed in 100 μl of TE buffer (10 mM Tris-HCl, 1 mM EDTA, pH 8.0) and DNA was eluted by incubation at 60°C for 3 h. To confirm that each band was differentially amplified and homogeneous, recovered DNA was amplified by the asymmetric PCR and subjected to the SSCP analysis. Residual dNTPs and the primers were removed using a spin filtration column (Suprec-02, Takara, Kyoto, Japan). Nucleotide sequences of amplified single stranded cDNA were determined by the dideoxy chain termination method using a modified T7 DNA polymerase (Sequenase version 2.0 kit, United States Biochemical, Cleveland, OH, USA) with the sequencing primers.

We carried out the sensitivity study on the SSCP analysis. A minor sequence consisting of 5% of the major sequence could be detected as a discrete band by the SSCP analysis, indicating that the SSCP method can detect quasispecies that occupy more than 5% of the whole HCV population. Theoretically, quasispecies that occupy more than 5% could be detected using the cloning-sequencing method by selecting 20 clones, but it should be emphasized again that there are millions of clones in the serum, and selection of 20 clones from millions is far from representative of the whole population.

General application

Four patients with chronic active hepatitis and HCV infection were studied. They had elevated serum transferase levels for more than six months. cDNA fragments containing the HVR were amplified from plasma RNA using PCR. PCR products were separated by the SSCP analysis. DNA fragments were recovered from SSCP bands in the gel, and their nucleotide sequences were determined. The SSCP analysis separated PCR products into several bands with different mobility. Sequence analysis of these bands confirmed that the

HCV populations in each patient are composed of quasispecies with different HVR. Different patterns of variation in the HVR quasispecies were observed in individual patients with different clinical features during chronic infection. In interferon treatment, some quasispecies disappeared during the treatment and reappeared after the end of the treatment, while other quasispecies in the same patient remained during the treatment, suggesting that the sensitivity to interferon is different among quasispecies. These results suggest that HCV populations fluctuate during the course of chronic infection and interferon treatment, suggesting that the intraisolate heterogeneity of HCV genome is associated with persistent infection and with resistance to interferon [20].

Mechanisms for appearance of HCV variants in chronic infection

To investigate further genetic backgrounds of the change in the HVR, plasma samples serially obtained from patients with chronic hepatitis C were studied [21]. The envelope gene containing the HVR was amplified and examined by the SSCP analysis. Furthermore, sequences of the quasispecies separated by the SSCP analysis were determined, and phylogenetic analyses were performed using the neighbor joining method. HCV populations within each individual were composed of several quasispecies. These quasispecies populations in vivo changed serially in most of the patients. Gradual selection of coexisting quasispecies was observed over 6 to 18 months in some patients, whereas complete replacements of previous quasispecies by new quasispecies were repeatedly observed at intervals of a few months in other patients. Phylogenetic analyses on these quasispecies revealed the continuous accumulation of mutations in some patients and discontinuous appearance of evolutionarily distant quasispecies in the other patient.

These results indicate that HCV quasispecies populations change during the natural course of chronic infection and these changes in the HVR of HCV genomes appear to be both continuous accumulation of mutations and selection of pre-existing minor variants from the large spectrum of quasispecies populations.

Host-dependent variations of HCV

Nucleotide sequences of envelope regions containing a part of the E1 gene and the HVR of HCV were determined after separating each HCV quasispecies by the SSCP analysis in patients in whom intrafamilial transmission of HCV was suspected. Populations of HCV genomes were composed of plural quasispecies in some patients, while they were composed of a single quasispecies in the others. Phylogenetic analysis on those quasispecies demonstrated that all quasispecies in each individual were highly homologous with each other. The homology was higher in the part of the E1 gene than the

HVR. Furthermore, all quasispecies found in the members of one family (husband and wife) were also highly homologous, suggesting direct intrafamilial transmission. Nevertheless, there were no common substitutions of nucleotide among these quasispecies. These findings suggest that the direction of HCV evolution in the HVR are different depending on the host (unpublished data).

Diversity of HCV quasispecies and its clinical significance

The relationship between the diversity of HVR quasispecies and the disease stage including chronic hepatitis, liver cirrhosis, and hepatocellular carcinoma has not been clarified. Furthermore, the relationship between the diversity of HVR quasispecies and the IFN responsiveness is not known. HCV quasispecies populations were separated in patients with chronic active hepatitis, liver cirrhosis, and hepatocellular carcinoma by the SSCP method targeted to the HVR (unpublished data).

Patients with multiple bands had significantly more progressed liver disease than those with a single band group. The ratio of patients with a single band was 36% in chronic active hepatitis and 0% in hepatocellular carcinoma. Among patients with chronic active hepatitis, those who had multiple bands were more resistant to IFN therapy than those who had a single band. Thus, the diversity of HVR quasispecies becomes more complex as the disease stage progresses. Patients with chronic active hepatitis who have complex diversity seem to be resistant to IFN treatment.

Comparison of the HVR of HCV genomes in the plasma and the liver

Nucleotide sequences of the HVR of HCV genomes obtained from plasma quickly change during the course of infection. It is not known, however, whether these changes also occur in the liver. To clarify this, RNA was extracted from the plasma and the liver tissue of patients with chronic hepatitis C. DNA fragments that included the HVR were amplified and consensus nucleotide sequences were directly determined from the PCR products by the dideoxy chain termination method. The diversity of the HVR was further analyzed by the SSCP analysis.

Consensus nucleotide sequences of the HVR were identical between the plasma and the liver in each patient. The SSCP analysis showed multiple DNA bands that represented different HVR sequences. Comparison of the SSCP patterns revealed that the number, the mobility, and the density of bands were identical between the plasma and the liver. The population and the diversity of HCV quasispecies as detected by the HVR sequence are identical between the plasma and the liver despite of its rapid mutations, indicating that rapid changes in the population of HCV quasispecies also occur in the liver [22].

Analysis of HCV quasispecies in hepatocellular carcinoma tissues

Although persistent HCV infection is closely related with the development of HCC, replication of HCV in HCC tissues has not been characterized. To study this, carcinoma and noncarcinoma tissues were obtained from patients with HCC. Total RNA was recovered from each tissue, and a part of the envelope gene of replicating HCV was amplified by the minus-strand specific RT-PCR. The amplified cDNA was examined by the SSCP analysis and sequencing.

Replicating HCV was detected in both carcinoma and noncarcinoma tissues in some patients who were positive for serum HCV markers. In some patients, the replicating HCV existed as a mixture of several quasispecies. In the other patient, a single quasispecies was obtained from both carcinoma and noncarcinoma tissues. The constitution of viral populations was different between carcinoma and noncarcinoma tissues. The difference in the constitution of quasispecies populations between carcinoma and noncarcinoma tissues confirms the unequivocal replication of HCV in both tissues, and may imply the presence of different biological properties among HCV with different sequences [23].

Changes in HCV quasispecies populations during IFN treatment

Mechanisms of IFN resistance have not been elucidated. As stated above, the degree of heterogeneity of HCV quasispecies in vivo appears to correlate with the resistance to IFN therapy. HCV quasispecies after IFN therapy are not similar to those before IFN. These observations suggest that some HCV quasispecies may be more resistant to IFN therapy than others. In order to evaluate the difference in IFN sensitivity among HCV quasispecies, analyses of serial changes in HCV quasispecies populations during IFN treatment in some individuals may provide useful information. Therefore, the fluctuation of HCV quasispecies was investigated by the SSCP analysis in patients who did not respond to IFN therapy and remained viremic during the treatment.

In all patients, the constitution of HCV quasispecies populations changed after the start of IFN therapy. In some patients, some of the HCV quasispecies coexisting before the IFN therapy were selected for and became predominant during the therapy, thereas the other quasispecies disappeared. In the other patient, new HCV quasispecies that had not been detected before the IFN therapy appeared and overwhelmed the pretreatment HCV during the IFN therapy. Moreover, in some patients, the predominant HCV quasispecies returned to the pretreatment virus after the cessation of IFN. In contrast, no significant changes were observed during the pretreatment period, implying that the changes in HCV quasispecies populations were closely associated with the IFN treatment. In some cases, deduced amino acid sequences of the HVR were identical between IFN-sensitive and IFN-resistant

HCV despite the difference in nucleotide sequences, indicating that immune responses to the HVR are not the determining factor of IFN sensitivity.

Thus, the sensitivity to IFN is different among HCV quasispecies, suggesting the existence of the IFN-resistant HCV strain. Since HCV quasispecies with identical amino acid sequences in the HVR respond differently to IFN, regions other than the HVR are important determinants for IFN resistance. Mechanisms of IFN resistance could be revealed by the analysis of the whole genome of IFN-resistant HCV (unpublished data).

Analysis of the whole genome of IFN-resistant HCV

The whole genome of a hepatitis C virus (HCV) genotype 1b with different sensitivity to interferon was studied in the same individuals to determine the genetic basis of their resistance. Comparative nucleotide sequence analysis of the whole genome from three pairs of sensitive and resistant HCV isolates identified the cluster of amino acid differences in the NS5 region. Additional sequence data of the NS5 region obtained from interferon-resistant HCV and interferon-sensitive HCV confirmed the exclusive existence of missense mutations in this interferon sensitivity determining region (ISDR). On the other hand, interferon-resistant HCV from interferon nonresponders had an ISDR identical to that of prototype HCV-1b. These results indicated that HCV-1b with prototype-ISDR is an interferon-resistant strain. The specific nature of these mutations would make it possible to develop the assays to predict interferon resistance (unpublished data).

References

1. Weiner AJ, Brauer MJ, Rosenblatt J et al. Virology 1991;180:842–848.
2. Hijikata M, Kato N, Ootsuyama Y et al. Biochem Biophys Res Commun 1991;175:220–228.
3. Kato N, Ootsuyama Y, Tanaka T et al. Virus Research 1992;22:107–123.
4. Kato N, Ootsuyama Y, Ohkoshi S et al. Biochem Biophys Res Commun 1992;189:119–127.
5. Ogata N, Alter HJ, Miller RH et al. Proc Natl Acad Sci USA 1991;88:3392–3396.
6. Weiner AJ, Geysen HM, Christopherson C et al. Proc Natl Acad Sci USA 1992;89:3468–3472.
7. Weiland E, Stark R, Haas B et al. J Virol 1990;64:3563–3569.
8. Rusche JR, Javaherian K, McDanal C et al. Proc Natl Sci Acad USA 1988;85:3198–3202.
9. Takahashi H, Cohen J, Hosmalin A et al. Proc Natl Acad Sci USA 1988;85:3105–3109.
10. Chomczynski P, Sacchi N. Anal Biochem 1987;162:156–159.
11. Saiki RK, Gelfand DH, Stoffel S et al. Science 1988;239:487–491.
12. Sakamoto N, Enomoto N, Kurosaki M et al. J Med Virol 1994;42:103–108.
13. Kurosaki M, Enomoto N, Marumo F et al. Hepatology 1993;18:1293–1299.
14. Okada S, Akahane Y, Suzuki H et al. Hepatology 1992;16:619–624.
15. Enomoto N, Sato C, Kurosaki M et al. J Hepatol 1994;20:252–261.
16. Martell M, Esteban JI, Quer J et al. J Virol 1992;66:3225–3229.
17. Holland JJ, De La Torre JC, Steinhauer DA. Current Topics in Microbiology and Immunology 1992;176:1–20.

18. Orita M, Suzuki Y, Sekiya T et al. Genomics 1989;5:874–879.
19. Yap EP-H, Lo Y-MD, Cooper K et al. Lancet 1992;340:736.
20. Enomoto N, Kurosaki M, Marumo F et al. J Gen Virol 1994;75:1361–1369.
21. Kurosaki M, Enomoto N, Marumo F et al. Virology 1994;206:161–169.
22. Sakamoto N, Enomoto N, Kurosaki M et al. Comparison of the hypervariable region of hepatitis C genomes in the plasma and the liver. J. Med Virol (in press).
23. Kurosaki M, Enomoto N, Hoshino Y et al. Detection and analysis of replicating hepatitis C virus quasispecies in hepatocellular carcinoma tissue. J Hepatol (in press).

Progress in Hepatology Vol. 1.
Cellular and Molecular Biology.
M. Yamanaka, K. Okabe and G. Toda, editors.

The present status of autoimmune hepatitis and its heterogeneity

Mikio Zeniya, Akira Kuramoto, Hiroki Takahashi, Yoshio Aizawa and Gotaro Toda
Department of Internal Medicine (I), The JIKEI University School of Medicine, Tokyo, Japan

Abstract. Owing to the recent discovery of clinical detection system for hepatitis C virus, the disease entity of autoimmune hepatitis has been clearly established. However, there are still no pathogmonic features of autoimmune hepatitis, and the diagnosis of this disease requires the exclusion of several liver diseases including viral infection. The autoantibodies associated with autoimmune hepatitis are neither pathogenic nor disease specific, we have not yet obtained autoimmune hepatitis-specific autoantibodies. Recently, several reports have indicated that autoantibodies and antibodies to hepatitis C virus with positive for serum HCV-RNA may occur together in patients who were diagnosed as autoimmune hepatitis.

The aim of this review is to define the heterogeneity of autoimmune hepatitis at present.

Key words: autoimmune hepatitis (AIH), HLA, hepatitis C virus (HCV), T cell receptor (TCR).

Introduction

Autoimmune hepatitis is an immunological disorder and an important cause of progressive necroinflammatory liver disease [1–4]. The common characteristics of this disorder include a female gender predominance, polyclonal hypergammaglobulinemia, the presence of circulating autoantibodies, and a generally favorable response to corticosteroid treatment [5,6]. However, it is also clear that there are immunologic, immunogenetic, histologic, geographic, and clinical heterogeneities among autoimmune hepatitis patients [7,8]. In the present study, we survey the current state of knowledge about the heterogeneity of autoimmune hepatitis, and present recent data on this subject collected by our department.

Heterogeneity of autoimmune hepatitis

Immunogenetic heterogeneity

Like other autoimmune diseases, autoimmune hepatitis is clearly associated with the human leucocytes antigen (HLA) haplotypes [9–12]. In the United

Address for correspondence: Mikio Zeniya, M.D., Department of Internal Medicine (I), The JIKEI University School of Medicine, 3-25-8, Nishi-Shinbashi, Minato, Tokyo 105, Japan. Tel: 81-3-3433-1111. Fax: 81-3-3435-0569.

Table 1. The result of HLA typing in 22 Japanese autoimmune hepatitis patients

			HLA											
Case	Sex	Age	A		B		C_w		DR_w		DR		DQ	
S.K.	F	25	**24**	–	35	61	–	–	53	–	**4**	9	3	**4**
T.K.	F	40	2	**24**	54	–	1	–	53	–	2	**4**	1	3
T.T.	F	59	33	–	39	67	7	–	53	–	1	**4**	1	3
K.K.	M	40	**24**	26	35	**52**	3	–	53	–	**4**	–	**4**	–
T.F.	F	44	2	**24**	35	39	3	7	53	–	**4**	–	1	**4**
S.Y.	F	50	2	–	35	60	3	–	53	–	**4**	9	3	–
C.E.	F	50	2	11	54	62	1	–	53	–	**4**	–	**4**	–
Y.K.	F	47	2	24	60	61	3	–	52	53	**4**	8	1	**4**
T.Y.	M	41	**24**	33	44	48	–	–	53	–	**4**	6	1	3
K.F.	F	49	**24**	26	**52**	67	1	–	53	–	2	**4**	1	**4**
H.K.	F	36	26	31	60	67	7	–	53	52	**4**	8	1	**4**
K.A.	F	54	2	**24**	52	61	–	–	53	–	2	**4**	1	**4**
F.H.	F	45	11	**24**	44	54	1	–	53	52	**4**	6	1	**4**
T.S.	F	55	2	26	46	54	1	3	52	53	**4**	6	1	**4**
Y.Y.	F	28	**24**	–	48	–	1	–	52	53	**4**	6	1	**4**
M.Y.	M	43	**24**	–	54	–	1	–	52	53	**4**	6	1	3
R.M.	M	67	3	31	51	59	7	–	53	–	2	**4**	1	3
S.I.	F	40	2	**24**	59	60	1	3	52	53	**4**	8	1	**4**
K.Y.	F	67	**24**	26	**52**	60	7	–	53	–	2	**4**	1	**4**
Y.M.	F	58	**24**	26	55	60	1	3	52	53	**4**	5	3	–
N.E.	F	54	**24**	–	46	**52**	1	–	52	–	2	5	1	3
N.Y.	M	64	2	–	35	61	3	–	52	–	2	9	1	3

Kingdom [13], Australia [14], North America [15–17], and probably continental Europe, HLA-A1-B8-DR3 is the disease-specific HLA haplotype, and HLA-DR3 is known as an important factor for susceptibility to autoimmune hepatitis. However, HLA-DR3 is less common in Asia, especially in Japan. In Asia, the frequency of HLA-DR3 in cases diagnosed as autoimmune hepatitis is less than 1% [18]. In Japan, autoimmune hepatitis is most strongly associated with HLA-DR4.

Despite this difference, clinical features of autoimmune hepatitis are similar regardless of geographic location. Recently, for example, HLA-DR4 was found to be a second risk factor for autoimmune hepatitis in the United Kingdom [13], and HLA-DR4-positive patients presented clinical signs at an older age and experienced a milder course of disease. These characteristics are similar to typical cases reported in Japan. HLA-DR3 and -DR4 appear to operate independently of one another in the genetic pathogenesis of autoimmune hepatitis. HLA-DR4 is the global immunogenetic factor that is not country specific of autoimmune hepatitis patients who showed mild clinical manifestation at a relatively older age.

Table 1 shows our HLA analysis for 22 recently diagnosed autoimmune

Table 2. HLA antigen freqencies in AIH patients and 60 area-matched Japanese controls. The frequencies of HLA-DR4 and HLA-DQ4 were significantly higher in the autoimmune hepatitis patients than in the sex- and age-matched normal controls The linkage of HLA-A24-B52-DR4-DQ4 was highly observed in Japanese autoimmune hepatitis patients

HLA	Control (n = 60)	Autoimmune hepatitis patients (n = 22)	χ^2	χ^2(c)	Corrected P value
A24	35	15	0.656	0.308	NS
B52	13	5	0.011	0.039	NS
B54	10	5	0.396	0.094	NS
DR2	19	7	0.0001	0.005	NS
DR4	24	20	16.778	14.793	<0.01
DQ4	9	13	15.940	13.774	<0.01
A24-B52	13	5	0.011	0.039	NS
B52-DR4	3	4	3.582	2.093	NS
DR4-DQ4	8	13	17.692	15.371	<0.01
B52-DR4-DQ4	1	4	7.668	5.055	<0.05
A24-B52-DR4-DQ4	1	4	7.668	5.055	<0.05

χ^2(c): corrected χ^2.

hepatitis patients from the Tokyo metropolitan area. Of the 22 subjects, five were male and 17 were female. The average age of the subjects was 49.1 years. We found no significant distribution of HLA class I antigens. Regarding HLA class II antigens, we found that the frequency of HLA-DR4 and HLA-DQ4 was significantly higher in the autoimmune hepatitis group than in our sex- and age-matched controls ($p < 0.01$). Furthermore, HLA-DR4 is a more significant genetic factor than HLA-DQ4 (χ^2 = 16.8 vs. 15.9, chi-square test) (Table 2), determining susceptibility to autoimmune hepatitis among the Japanese. We also found that all patients who did not have HLA-DR4 did have HLA-DR2, and were older than the patients who had HLA-DR4. Seki et al. [19] reported the same results in his HLA analysis of Japanese autoimmune hepatitis, indicating HLA-DR2 may be another genetic factor in Japanese autoimmune hepatitis. There were no other clinical differences between HLA-DR2-positive and -DR4-positive patients. The patients who showed both HLA-DR4 and -DR2 also showed similar clinical manifestations (unpublished data).

Our study of 22 patients found that the presence of the specific haplotype, HLA-A24-B52-DR4-DQ4, was significant in autoimmune hepatitis ($p < 0.05$). The high incidence of HLA-DQ4 may be explained by the existence of a strong disequilibrium between HLA-DR4 and HLA-DQ4 in Japanese patients. We also found that the serum level of transaminase at onset is much higher in the haplotype-positive group than in the haplotype-negative group,

Table 3. HLA types and clinical features (age of onset and maximum serum ALT level) in DR4-positive autoimmune hepatitis patients. The patients with HLA A24-B52-DR4-DQ4 showed an older onset and higher maximum serum ALT levels than those without this haplotype, however these differences were not statistically significant

HLA	n	Age (y)	Max. ALT (mU/ml)
DQ4 (+)	13	45.0 ± 3.1	500.8 ± 143.2
DQ4 (−)	7	51.1 ± 3.7	386.9 ± 132.6
A24-B52-DR4-DQ4 (+)	4	52.5 ± 4.9	923.8 ± 325.0
A24-B52-DR4-DQ4 (−)	16	45.8 ± 2.7	376.4 ± 78.0

Table 4. HLA antigens and the efficacy of corticosteroid therapy in DR4-positive autoimmune hepatitis patients. Eighteen of the 20 autoimmune hepatitis patients achieved complete remission, and 6 relapsed. A24-B52-DR4-DQ4-positive patients showed significantly higher relapse rates than A24-B52-DR4-DQ4-negative patients ($p < 0.05$)

HLA	Autoimmune hepatitis patients (n = 20)	Remission at 6 months (n = 18)	Relapse after remission (n = 6)
DQ4 (+)	13	11	4
DQ4 (−)	7	7	2
A24-B52-DR4-DQ4 (+)	4	4	4*
A24-B52-DR4-DQ4 (−)	16	14	2*

*, $p < 0.05$.

and that the recurrence rate after immunosuppressive therapy was also high in the haplotype-positive group (Tables 3 and 4). This result suggests that the DQ4 haplotype may be related to the maintenance or worsening of autoimmune hepatitis. However, the number of the patients who had HLA-A24-B52-DR4-DQ4 was not large. Further analysis is needed.

In the HLA class II loci, there are 3 major class II subregions, DR, DQ, and DP, each of which contains several genes. It has been reported that there is a nonpolymeric DRA gene, the product of which can form a dimer with the product of each of the four expressed DRB genes, namely, DRB1, DRB3, DRB4, and DRB5, in the DR subregion. The DRB1 gene is highly polymorphic and codes for the serologically defined series of DR epitopes. The DRB4 gene is, in contrast, nonpolymorphic, and the DRA-DRB4 dimer is expressed on DR4, DR7, and DR9 haplotypes. The DRB5 gene has 4 different alleles occurring on different DR2 haplotypes [20]. Recently, specific amino acid sequences of polymorphic HLA antigens have been suggested as contributing to the susceptibility and resistance of individuals to autoimmune disease [21]. Polymorphic HLA-DRB1 and/or DQB1 molecules are reported

Table 5. The frequency of DR4-derived DRβ1 alleles in 18 patients with HLA-DR4-positive autoimmune hepatitis. Frequencies of normal Japanese HLA-DR4-derived DRβ1 alleles were reported in [32]

Allele	Dw type	Number of autoimmune hepatitis patients (%)	Number of Japanese controls (%)	Relative risk
0401	4	1(5.6)	3(4.7)	1.19
0403	13a	1(5.6)	9(13.8)	0.41
0405	115	14(77.8)	41(63.1)	1.23
0406	KT2	2(11.1)	8(12.3)	0.90
0407	13b	0(0)	2(3.1)	–
0408	14b	0(0)	2(3.1)	–

to influence the development of several autoimmune diseases, such as rheumatoid arthritis [22], insulin-dependent diabetes mellitus [23,24], celiac disease [25], and pemphigus vulgaris [26].

We amplified the DRβ gene using the PCR technique, using the DNA extracted from peripheral mononuclear cells of our patients. We then analyzed the DR4 genotype using the sequence-specific oligonucleotide method [27] and restriction fragment length polymorphism, using genotype-specific oligonucleotides as probes [28,29]. Table 5 shows our analysis of the HLA-DRB1 molecules in our autoimmune hepatitis patients. The results showed that the frequency of the 0105 allele was high in autoimmune hepatitis (77.8%). However, the frequency of the same allele in normal Japanese controls was also high, up to 63%. This indicates that there are no autoimmune hepatitis-specific alleles in Japanese patients. There may be unknown specific amino acid sequences common in DR4 but not common in other HLA-DRs.

Immunological heterogeneity

Early works in this area indicated that the presence of LE cell phenomenon was one of the most important features of autoimmune hepatitis [30]. At present, it is clear that only a minority of autoimmune hepatitis patients, probably 10–15% or less, test positive for LE cells [31]. In Japan, LE cell-positive autoimmune patients are diagnosed as having typical autoimmune hepatitis, called lupoid hepatitis in the original articles [32]. However, such patients do not always present distinctive clinical or histological features [31–33].

The antinuclear antibody is one of the most important diagnostic factors for autoimmune hepatitis [34,35]. Though the presence of antinuclear antibody

Table 6. Differences of clinical manifestation between prototype autoimmune hepatitis and HCV-related autoimmune hepatitis

	Prototype autoimmune hepatitis	HCV-related autoimmune hepatitis
Number of cases	17	15
Male or female	3/14	4/11
Average age	47.1	52.6
Positive rate	17/17(100%)	15/15(100%)
ANA titer (median)	160–10,240(640**)	40–640(80)
Positive rate of ASMA	5/14(35.2%)	4/15(26.7%)
Positive rate of LE test	3/14(28.6%)	2/11(18.2%)
AST (mean ± SD)	496.6 ± 352.0	201.0 ± 88.4*
ALT (mean ± SD)	557.7 ± 482.3	219.0 ± 121.1**
IgG (mean ± SD)	3,125.5 ± 681.3	3,205.2 ± 421.5
DR4-positive	17/17(100%)	9/15(60%)
Initial steroid effect	14/14(100%)	7/7(100%)
Remission at 6 months	14/14(100%)	6/7(85.7%)
Relapse	4/14(28.6%)	2/7(28.6%)
Remission at 2 years	9/14(64.3%)	2/7(28.6%)

*$p < 0.01$, **$p < 0.05$.

was detected originally using an indirect immunofluorescent technique using rodent tissue, most laboratories now use an established cell line, such as Hep-2 cells for the detection of antinuclear antibody. This creates some confusion in the diagnosis of autoimmune hepatitis. The assay for antinuclear antibody using Hep-2 cells is more sensitive than that using rodent tissue. Thus 30–40% of chronic hepatitis cases, especially in chronic hepatitis C, tested positive for antinuclear antibody [36–38]. The titer of antinuclear antibody in chronic viral hepatitis is usually low, below 80×, but there are patients who show a high titer antinuclear antibody (over 160×). The chronic hepatitis of these patients cannot be differentiated from typical autoimmune hepatitis [39] (Table 6).

The problem of whether to include this virus-associated autoimmune reaction as a subset of autoimmune hepatitis remains to be resolved. In some cases, antinuclear antibody-positive virus-associated autoimmune hepatitis responds well to an initial corticosteroid therapy [40]. At present, it seems likely that these cases, especially those involving chronic hepatitis C, are best excluded from consideration as "ordinary" hepatitis C cases, in which interferon therapy is indicated [41].

By immunofluorescent technique, most of our antinuclear antibody-positive cases showed a similar – homogeneous – staining pattern to cases of systemic lupus erythematosus, in which the reactivity of the antibody is clearly directed to double-strand DNA. In autoimmune hepatitis the antibodies to double-strand DNA are seldom detected by a specific assay [42–44]. These patterns may be helpful for diagnosis. We note, however, that antinuclear antibodies are a heterogeneous group of antibodies [42,45,46], and that these antibodies are found in other liver diseases.

High titers of IgG class anti-smooth muscle antibodies with antiactin specificity are also considered to be associated with autoimmune hepatitis. However, high titers of this antibody have been reported in primary biliary cirrhosis. In addition, only 52% of high titer IgG-type, anti-smooth muscle antibody reacts with actin in autoimmune hepatitis.

Subtypes of autoimmune hepatitis by autoantibodies

The presence of other autoantibodies, and the subdivision of autoimmune hepatitis by specific autoantibodies, has been reported [47,48]. Three subdivisions of autoimmune hepatitis have been reported on the basis of autoantibodies [49–52]. A fourth subdivision, in which the patients lack any of the conventional immunoserologic markers, is also justified [50].

The most prevalent subcategory of autoimmune hepatitis, prototype or classic autoimmune hepatitis (type I), is characterized by the presence of antinuclear and antiactin antibodies. A second subgroup (type II) is characterized by the presence of anti-liver-kidney microsomal (anti-LKM) antibody and the absence of antinuclear antibody [53]. Most of the patients diagnosed as type II were of younger age and showed rapid progression [54,55]. In the United States, only 4% of autoimmune hepatitis patients were categorized as type II [56]. Some hepatitis C virus (HCV)-positive patients also tested positive for anti-LKM antibody [57–60], and this group is currently classified as a second subgroup of type II autoimmune hepatitis. The existence of this HCV-positive and anti-LKM-positive autoimmune hepatitis introduced some controversies, in that it may allow the existence of viral-originated autoimmune hepatitis. In Japan, where the frequency of HCV-positivity is much higher than in Western countries, very few anti-LKM antibody-positive cases were detected [32], adding to the controversy. If HCV infection can induce anti-LKM-positive autoimmune hepatitis, there should be a high frequency of both HCV-positive and anti-LKM antibody-positive cases in Japan. A positive response to the anti-LKM antibody may relate to genetic susceptibility, particularly in HLA-DR3-positive patients, and it may be possible to induce anti-LKM antibody-positive autoimmune hepatitis under HCV infection. Further worldwide analysis of additional data will be needed to answer this question.

The third group of autoimmune hepatitis tests positive for the antisoluble liver antibody [52,61]. This antibody reacts against hepatocytic cytokeratins 8 and 18 [51], and was found only in patients with autoimmune hepatitis type III. Patients with type III autoimmune hepatitis were found to have many characteristics of the type I disease [62], such as a predominance in middle-aged females. However, they lacked antibodies to nuclear antigen, LKM antigen, and thyroid-related antigens. Of this group, 35% of patients were seropositive for smooth-muscle antibodies, and 26% showed antibodies to liver membrane antigen. Additionally, 22% of the patients were seropositive for antimitochondrial antibodies [60,61]. At present, type III autoimmune hepatitis with antisoluble liver antigen may be an unusual variant of the prototype autoimmune hepatitis, rather than an independent subtype. These variations and overlaps in dividing autoimmune hepatitis into subcategories by autoantibodies indicate that this method may be of limited utility in a clinical setting.

Other candidate autoantibodies categorized in autoimmune hepatitis

Asialoglycoprotein receptor is a receptor on the hepatic membrane and participates in the binding and endocytosis of serum asialoglycoproteins bearing terminal galactose or residues of N-acetyl-galactosamine [63,64]. It is distinct from other carbohydrate receptors, and specificity for hepatocyte has been confirmed by biochemical and electron microscopic autoradiographic analysis [65,66]. It has been reported that the antiasialoglycoprotein receptor antibody is the specific autoantibody for autoimmune hepatitis in Western countries [67–70]. Titers of this antibody strongly correlated with histologic activity, but not with serum IgG levels, or with titers of other autoantibodies. Furthermore, after complete remission from immunosuppressive therapy, this autoantibody disappeared from some patients with autoimmune hepatitis [70]. To complicate matters, this antibody was also found in the case of primary biliary cirrhosis and chronic viral hepatitis [70]. In Japan, this autoantibody was found in most autoimmune hepatitis patients. The disease specificity of this antibody is still unclear.

Toda et al. reported that sera from autoimmune hepatitis patients reacted against hepatocyte plasma membrane [71]. They found that the acidic glycolipid fraction of rabbit hepatocyte plasma membrane reacted with the serum from autoimmune hepatitis patients, and identified the target antigen for this antibody as sulfatide, a glycolipid [72,73]. The antibody to sulfatide was detected by enzyme-linked immunosorbent assay (ELISA) and was found to be specific for autoimmune hepatitis. Unfortunately, sulfatide is not liver specific. It is primarily observed in brain tissue and is relatively scarce in the liver. The antibody may also react with sulfate-sulfatide. The presence of heparin diminished the antibody activity by 90% in the ELISA assay, whereas keratan sulfate, chondroitin sulfate type A and C and dermatan sulfate did not diminish activity even at high concentration [72]. These data indicated that the antisulfatide antibody cross-reacted with heparin. Endothelial cells possess a heparin-like structure on the surface, indicating that this antisulfatide antibody reacts with hepatic sinusoidal endothelial cells through this heparin-like structure. The same research group reported a significant increase in the IgG fraction of antisulfatide antibody bound to sinusoidal endothelial cells observed in autoimmune hepatitis [72,73]. Thus, the antibody to sinusoidal cells might be involved in the development and perpetuation of immunological hepatocyte injury in autoimmune hepatitis.

Hepatitis virus and autoimmune hepatitis

Antibodies to bacteria, such as *Escherichia coli*, *Bacteroid*, and *Salmonella*, and to nonhepatitis viral agents, such as measles, rubella, and cytomegalovirus, have been ascribed etiologic importance in autoimmune hepatitis [74–76]. A damaged liver may be unable to sequester exogenous antigen properly, and such infection could result in the alteration of the antibody formation pathway. Thus a genetically restricted host-dependent immunological response could be altered by infections. The viral nature of autoimmune hepatitis was first reported in the mid-1960s. No hepatitis virus had been discovered at that time, and no viral agent causing autoimmune hepatitis has since been reported. The measles virus genome has been found in peripheral lymphocytes in autoimmune hepatitis cases [77], indicating that measles virus may be an etiologic agent in some patients. However, a similar phenomenon has been reported in some patients with systemic lupus erythematosus, rheumatoid arthritis, and cryptogenic cirrhosis [78]. These observations may be an epiphenomenon, or a measles virus infection may stimulate an autoimmune reaction.

After the discovery of the hepatitis B virus, it was reported that lupus erythematosus cells were present in 10% of these cases. However, this phenomenon was regarded as a by-product of infection, and such autoimmunologic features were thought to be minimal [79–81]. According to a study by a Japanese health and welfare group, no hepatitis B-infected patient could be diagnosed with autoimmune hepatitis. This study concluded that there was no hepatitis B-related autoimmune hepatitis.

There is some evidence of a viral cause of autoimmune hepatitis, based on the results of surveys that have screened patients with autoimmune hepatitis for anti-HCV antibody [82–85]. A number of patients with autoimmune hepatitis tested positive for the anti-HCV antibody. In the early reports, however, many of the tests for anti-HCV antibody were not confirmed by subsequent RIBA and/or HCV-RNA tests [86,87]. Yet, there were autoimmune hepatitis patients who showed clear HCV infection [40]. Unfortunately, the pathogenetic relationship between an HCV infection and autoimmune hepatitis is uncertain. Because autoantibodies are neither pathogenetic nor disease specific, it is uncertain whether HCV is an immunogenetic stimulus or if it triggers a cellular cytotoxicity against viral infected hepatocytes.

We are unaware of any animal experiments of viral infection which have not been complicated by autoimmune hepatitis. Yet there are only a few cases of human patients treated with interferon who develop autoimmune hepatitis, despite the emergence of high titers of autoantibodies. Viral infection by itself may be an insufficient cause to induce autoimmune hepatitis. An idiosyncratic feature partly associated with genetic factors may be involved in the pathogenesis of HCV-associated autoimmune hepatitis.

Heterogeneity in treatment

Autoimmune hepatitis is characterized by a good response to corticosteroid. However, nearly 20% of patients show spontaneous remission [88]. This phenomenon suggested that some cases of autoimmune hepatitis may be induced by exposure to a common viral or environmental agent. It has been reported that a high frequency of antimeasles antibody was observed in many cases of autoimmune hepatitis [76–78]. Furthermore, natural remission is also described in chronic hepatitis C.

In a recent study, we reported that the initial response rate to corticosteroid is nearly 100% in HCV-related autoimmune hepatitis. However, after 2 years of follow-up, the rate of sustained remission is lower than in HCV-negative autoimmune hepatitis [40] (Table 6). This suggests that HCV infection may induce an autoimmune hepatitis-like disease condition, and that immunosuppressive therapy may have value in tracing this condition. Furthermore, successful interferon treatment was reported in HCV-positive autoimmune hepatitis. Autoimmune-related symptoms cleared up after treatment with eradicating serum HCV-RNA. This strongly suggests that there have been a few cases of HCV-related autoimmune hepatitis. It is also possible that HCV infection occurred incidentally in autoimmune hepatitis patients. However, these clinical insights remain conjectural.

Present status of autoimmune hepatitis in Japan

Diagnostic status

Table 7 shows the diagnostic criteria for autoimmune hepatitis recommended by a Japanese national study group in 1992 [32]. In these criteria there were several features compared to conventional criteria, one of which was described by Mackay [39]. Both erythrocyte sedimentation rate and serum value of C-reactive protein were listed as clinical indices for the diagnosis. Though these markers are not specific for autoimmune hepatitis, in most cases of viral-associated chronic hepatitis it is very rare that both tests show abnormal values.

Table 7. Criteria for diagnosis of autoimmune hepatitis in Japan. Study Group of Japanese Ministry of Health and Welfare, 1992

General concept

Increased prevalence in younger females, chronic active hepatitis with potential progression to cirrhosis, existence of autoimmune mechanisms in etiology, exclusion of all other known specific causes of chronic hepatitis, such as viruses, alcohol, drugs, etc, good response to corticosteroid therapy (typical).

I. Major findings
1. Persistent elevation of serum aminotransferases.
2. Hypergammaglobulinemia of 2.5 g/dl or greater (or IgG concentration of 2.5 g/dl or greater).
3. Circulating autoantibody: a) and/or b)
   a) LE test positive[1]
   b) ANA (antinuclear antibody) positive and/or LE test positive[2]
4. IgM anti-HAN (hepatitis A virus) negative and absence of other evidence of HBV infection (HBs antigen negative, antiHBc antibody negative or at low titers).
5. Absence of true-positive anti-HCV antibody or other evidence of HCV infection.

II. Minor findings
1. Systemic manifestation such as fever, arthralgia and skin eruption.
2. Complication of other autoimmune diseases including Collagen disease.[3]
3. a) and/or b)
   a) Accelerated ESR (erythrocyte sedimentation rate) at 30 mm/hr or faster.
   b) C-reactive protein (CRP) positive.

III. Histology

Chronic active hepatitis or cirrhosis with marked plasma cell infiltration and hepatocyte necrosis, absence of features of other specific diagnosis such as alfa-1-antitrypsin deficiency.[4]

Diagnosis of autoimmune hepatitis
1) Diagnostic: Fulfill all criteria of I and III.
2) Suggestive: Fulfill all criteria of I and at least one of II.
3) Possible: Fulfill all criteria of I.

[1]Autoimmune hepatitis with LE cell phenomenon also referred as "Lupoid hepatitis".
[2]Autoimmune hepatitis being positive for anti-liver-kidney-microsome 1 antibody but for which negative antinuclear antibody has been reported.
[3]Autoimmune hepatitis cases which need to be differentiated from SLE have to fulfill III and have to be negative for proteinuria.
[4]There may be some cases which are histologically acute hepatitis.

In the 1992 criteria, HCV infection is not completely excluded from the territory of autoimmune hepatitis. Furthermore, in a recent diagnostic index for autoimmune hepatitis proposed by the International Autoimmune Hepatitis Group, HCV infection was not excluded. In fact, there were some reports that indicated that HCV infection may be closely associated to the pathogenesis of autoimmune hepatitis. The term "autoimmune" seems interchangeable with "idiopathic" at present. This raised the question of whether the viral-associated autoimmune phenomena could be involved in the prototype autoimmune hepatitis. This question creates clinical problems, for when the diagnosis of autoimmune hepatitis is made in patients positive for HCV-RNA, it is difficult to decide which therapeutic regimen (corticosteroids or interferon) is best [89].

Recent advances in autoimmune hepatitis

Dramatic advances in the techniques of molecular biology have provided new tools for the clinical analysis of autoimmune mechanisms. The quantitative polymerase chain reaction established by Choi et al. [90], may serve well for the rapid estimation of human T cell repertoires, as there are limited numbers of monoclonal antibodies against at least 20 different Vβ families in humans [91]. We are now trying to examine the mechanism of autoimmunity in autoimmune hepatitis by analyzing the repertoire of T cell receptor (TCR) genes in both peripheral and liver-infiltrating lymphocytes [92]. A brief summary of our most recent work appears below.

T cell receptor analysis

Peripheral blood mononuclear cells and liver-infiltrating lymphocytes were obtained from six newly diagnosed autoimmune hepatitis patients before treatment with immunosuppressive agent. HLA typing was performed using a microcytotoxicity test. Peripheral blood mononuclear lymphocytes were separated using Ficoll-Hypaque density gradient centrifugation. Liver-infiltrating lymphocytes were obtained from liver biopsy specimens, which were minced and filtered through a metallic mesh, and the lymphocytes isolated using Ficoll-Hypaque centrifugation. Total RNA of about 3–10 μg was prepared by using RNA zol solution from both peripheral blood mononuclear cells and liver-infiltrating lymphocytes. cDNAs were synthesized in a 20 μl reaction mixture containing oligo (dT) primer by AMV reverse transcriptase from 5 μg of total RNA. Amplification was performed with Taq polymerase in 50 μl of standard buffer by different Vβ and Cβ primers as shown in Table 8.

Percent usage of TCR Vβ was calculated using the following methods. For quantification of TCR Vβ and Cβ gene transcripts, PCR products were separated using 5% polyacrylamide gel electrophoresis (PAGE) and the bands of PCR products were quantified using a densitometer (Fuji BAS2000, Fujifilm Co., Tokyo). Gels were scanned on a BAS2000 image analyzer (Fuji). The relative amounts of TCR Vβ and Cβ were calculated using standardization curves. The %Vβ usage was represented by Vβ/Cβ as

Table 8. Sequence of primers used for PCR

Primer	$5' \rightarrow 3'$ sequence
Vβ1	GCACAACAGTTCCCTGACTTGCAC
Vβ2	TCATCAACCATGCAAGCCTGACCT
Vβ3	GTCTCTAGAGAGAAGAAGGAGCGC
Vβ4	ACATATGAGAGTGGATTTGTCATT
Vβ5.1	ATACTTCAGTGAGACACAGAGAAAC
Vβ5.2	TTCCCTAACTATAGCTCTGAGCTG
Vβ6	AGGCCTGAGGGATCCGTCTC
Vβ7	CCTGAATGCCCCAACAGCTCTC
Vβ8	ATTTACTTTAACAACAACGTTCCG
Vβ9	CCTAAATCTCCAGACAAAGCTCAC
Vβ10	CTCCAAAAACTCATCCTGTACCTT
Vβ11	TACACAGTCTCCAGAATAAGGACG
Vβ12	AAAGGAGAAGTCTCAGAT
Vβ13.1	CAAGGAGAAGTCCCCAAT
Vβ13.2	GGTGAGGGTACAACTGCC
Vβ14	GTCTCTCGAAAAGAGAAGAGGAAT
Vβ15	AGTGTCTCTCGACAGGCACAGGCT
Vβ16	AAAGAGTCTAAACAGGATGAGTCC
Vβ17	CAGATAGTAAATGACTTTCAG
Vβ18	GATGAGTCAGGAATGCCAAAGGAA
Vβ19	CAATGCCCCAAGAACGCACCCTGC
Vβ20	AGCTCTGAGGTGCCCCAGAATCTC
3′Cβ	TTCTGATGGCTCAAACAC
5′Cα	GAACCCTGACCCTGCCGTGTACC
3′Cα	ATCATAAATTCGGGTAGGATCC

calculated using the formula,

$$\beta\%\mathrm{V(x)} = \frac{\dfrac{\mathrm{PSL\,V\beta(x)}}{\mathrm{PSL\,C\alpha(x)}}}{\sum^{1-22}\left(\dfrac{\mathrm{PSL\,V\beta}}{\mathrm{PSL\,C\alpha}}\right)} \times 100$$

Table 9 shows the result of our analysis on the usage of TCR Vβ in both peripheral blood lymphocytes and liver-infiltrating lymphocytes. Some TCR Vβ was predominantly used in liver tissue as compared to peripheral blood. The T cells expressing Vβ7, Vβ10, Vβ13.2, and Vβ19 in liver-infiltrating lymphocytes increased in number compared with the findings for peripheral blood lymphocytes. The amount of Vβ usage in liver-infiltrating lymphocytes was at least 1.5× more than that of peripheral blood lymphocytes. These results indicate that there are differences in Vβ usage in

Table 9. TCR Vβ gene expression of peripheral blood (PBL) and liver-infiltrating (LIL) lymphocytes in three autoimmune hepatitis patients.

Vβ	Mean ± 2SD* (%)	Percentage of expression: Autoimmune hepatitis patient 1		Autoimmune hepatitis patient 2		Autoimmune hepatitis patient 3	
		PBL	LIL	PBL	LIL	PBL	LIL
1	5.5 ± 3.45	6.6	5.2	2.5	11.3	5.1	19.8
2	8.4 ± 3.13	11.2	4.7	1.5	6.9	10.2	9.4
3	9.4 ± 2.14	8.3	4.2	1.9	12.0	7.7	12.4
4	7.4 ± 1.76	8.5	1.5	2.7	2.9	3.1	1.7
5.1	5.4 ± 2.92	6.3	2.0	4.9	2.9	4.6	2.1
5.2	3.4 ± 2.09	2.8	1.7	3.3	4.0	4.1	4.0
6	6.0 ± 4.1	7.0	7.4	1.8	6.8	6.1	7.7
7	8.5 ± 3.59	5.6	11.1	2.1	6.9	6.1	7.2
8	3.8 ± 1.52	3.0	2.1	6.0	3.1	4.1	3.0
9	4.7 ± 1.6	8.8	4.7	9.0	3.7	3.6	3.3
10	2.6 ± 0.89	2.3	4.7	8.3	3.2	3.1	0.8
11	2.4 ± 1.23	1.7	1.6	4.2	2.2	2.6	0.8
12	0.9 ± 1.27	0.9	1.2	6.6	3.0	2.0	1.7
13.1	3.0 ± 1.39	2.0	2.4	7.4	3.1	2.0	2.9
13.2	3.0 ± 1.88	2.6	8.0	4.3	3.1	7.1	3.9
14	6.0 ± 2.62	3.9	4.0	2.0	3.2	2.0	3.4
15	3.1 ± 0.92	4.0	4.2	5.5	3.3	4.1	5.6
16	2.4 ± 0.87	1.7	2.1	8.1	3.4	2.0	1.7
17	1.1 ± 0.97	1.2	1.6	4.8	4.2	1.5	1.2
18	3.4 ± 1.16	2.6	5.5	5.3	3.0	5.1	1.7
19	2.7 ± 1.47	4.4	13.0	4.0	3.6	5.6	2.9
20	2.5 ± 1.81	4.6	6.9	4.0	4.1	8.1	2.7

*TCR Vβ gene expression obtained from normal controls

liver-infiltrating T cells in autoimmune hepatitis. However, the TCR Vβs differed in each case, suggesting that there are no disease-specific differences in TCR Vβ.

We noticed a close association between Vβ usage of liver-infiltrating lymphocytes and HLA phenotypes. For example, in the cases where liver-infiltrating lymphocytes predominantly expressed Vβ1, HLA-B46 and -DR9 were common. In other cases where Vβ usage was predominantly Vβ7, HLA-A24 was in common (unpublished data).

In the single-strand conformation polymorphism (SSCP) analyses of our patients, we could not detect any well-defined bands, as seen in our controls, suggesting that the TCR Vβ chain did not clone extensively in autoimmune hepatitis. Similar tests performed on our patients' peripheral blood lymphocytes and liver-infiltrating lymphocytes gave the same results.

Table 10. The results of TCV Vβ sequencing

	Vβ7	N-D-N	Jβ	
Clone 1	GCCAGCAGCCAAGA	GGGTGGGCGG	TCCTACGAGCAGTACTTC	2.7
	AlaSerSer Gln Glu	Gly GlyArg	SerTyrGlu Gln TyrPhe	
Clone 2	GCCAGCAGCCAAGA	TGGCAGGAATACC	TACAATGAGCAGTTC	2.1
	AlaSer SerGln Asp	Gly ArgAsnThr	TyrAsnGlu Gln Phe	
Clone 3	GCCAGCAGCC	GGGGACTAGCACAC	ACAGATACGCAGTATTTT	2.3
	AlaSer SerArg	Gly LeuAla His	Thr AspThr GlnTyrPhe	
Clone 6	GCCAGCAGCCAAG	NGGGGGCT	AACTATGGCTACACC	1.2
	Ala SerSerGln ---	GlyAla	AsnTyr GlyTyrThr	
Clone 7	GCCAGCAGCCAAG	TTCGGGGNTCCCGCGAGGAGG	ACACTGAAGCTTTC	1.1
	Ala SerSerGln Val	ArgGly SerArgGluGlu Asp	Thr Glu AlaPhe	
Clone 8	GCCAGCAGCCAAG	GTGAGGGC	TCCTACAATGAGCAGTTC	2.1
	Ala Ser SerGlnGly	Glu Gly	SerTyrAsnGlu GlnPhe	
Clone 9	GCCAGCAGCCAAGA	GGGACTAGCGGGAG	ACGAGCAGTACTTC	2.7
	Ala Ser SerGlnGlu	Gly Leu AlaGlyAsp	Glu Gln TyrPhe	
Clone 10	GCCAGCAGCCAAGA	TGGCAAGGGCG	CCTACGAGCAGTACTTC	2.7
	Ala Ser SerGlnAsp	GlyLysGlyAla	TyrGlu Gln TyrPhe	

We are currently analyzing TCR Vβ sequencing to confirm the ability of liver-infiltrating lymphocytes to clone oligo in autoimmune hepatitis. Briefly, our methods are as follows. Amplified PCR products were ligated to the blunt end of pUC18, and JM109 cells were used as the competent cells. After obtaining plasmid DNA, the sequences were analyzed. The study is not yet complete, but we found that in case 5, six out of eight clones used Jβ2.7 in Vβ3 of liver-infiltrating lymphocytes and two clones used Jβ2.1. No other Jβ was utilized. Furthermore, the two clones which utilized Jβ2.1 showed the same sequences, suggesting the liver-infiltrating lymphocytes have at least some ability to clone (Table 10).

In the same cases, three clones utilizing Jβ2.7 and two clones utilizing Jβ2.1 were observed in Vβ7-expressed liver-infiltrating lymphocytes. In these Jβ chains, we observed common amino acid sequences, including glutamate-glutamate at the 5′ site. This result indicates that the relatively restricted Jβ chain of the TCRβ chain was utilized in the liver-infiltrating lymphocytes of the autoimmune hepatitis patients.

Summary

After the discovery of the assay system for hepatitis C infection, the clinical independence of autoimmune hepatitis was clearly established. In general, prototype autoimmune hepatitis is infrequently associated with viral hepatitis infection. However, there are occasionally patients with true viral infection, especially by HCV, and high titers of autoantibodies. In these patients, the treatment must be balanced for both the autoimmune disorder and the viral infection.

References

1. Mackay IR, Weiden S, Hasker J. Ann NY Acad Sci 1965;124:767–780.
2. Czaja AJ. In: Czaja AJ, Dickson ER (eds) Chronic Active Hepatitis, The Mayo Clinic Experience, New York: Decker, 1986;105–126.
3. Maddrey WC. In: Zakim D, Boyer TD (Eds) A Textbook of Liver disease, 2nd ed. Philadelphia: W.B. Saunders, 1990;1025–1061.
4. Mackay IR, Tait BT. In: Nishioka M, Toda G, Zeniya M (eds), Autoimmune Hepatitis, Amsterdam: Elsevier Science, 1994;3–23.
5. Czaja AJ. In: Krawitt EL, Wiesner RH (eds) Autoimmune Liver Diseases, New York: Raven Press, 1991;143–166.
6. Czaja AJ. In: Nishioka M, Toda G, Zeniya M (eds) Autoimmune Hepatitis, Amsterdam: Elsevier Science, 1994;27–43.
7. Johnson PJ, McFarlane IG, Eddleston ALWF. Sem Liver Dis 1991;11:187–196.
8. Zeniya M, Watanabe F, Aizawa Y et al. Gastroenterol Jap 1993;28(suppl):69–75.
9. Mackay IR, Morris PJ. Lancet 1976;II:793–795.
10. Tait BD, Mackay IR, Board P et al. Gastroenterology 1989;97:479–481.
11. Seki S, Kiyosawa K, Inoko H et al. Hepatology 1990;12:1300–1304.

12. Zeniya M, Takahashi H, Aoyama N et al. In: Tsuchiya M et al. (eds), Frontiers of Mucosal Immunology, vol. 2, Amsterdam: Excepta Medica, 1991;61–64.
13. Donaldson PT, Doherty DG, Hayllar KM et al. Hepatology 1991;13:701–706.
14. Mackay IR, Tait BD. Gastroenterology 1980;79:95–98.
15. Czaja AJ, Carpenter HA, Santrach PJ et al. Hepatology 1993;18:816–822.
16. Krawitt EL, Kilby AE, Albertini RJ et al. Hepatology 1987;7:1305–1310.
17. Tait BD, Mackay IR, Kastelan A et al. In: Terasaki FI (ed) Histocompatibility Testing 1980. UCLA Tissue Typing Laboratory, 1980;657–661.
18. Zeniya M, Watanabe F, Aizawa Y et al. In: Nishioka M, Toda G, Zeniya M (eds) Autoimmune Hepatitis, Amsterdam: Elsevier Science, 1994;267-279.
19. Seki T, Ota M, Furuta S et al. Gastroenterology 1992;103:1041–1047.
20. Bodmer JG, Marsh SGE, Albert ED et al. Tissue Antigens 1992;39:161–173.
21. Gregersen PK, Silver J, Wincheter RJ. Arthritis Rheum 1987;30:1205–1213.
22. Nepom GT, Hausen JA, Nepom BS. J Clin Immunol 1987;7:1–7.
23. Todd JA, Bell JI, McDevitt HO. Immunol Today 1988;4:129–134.
24. Baisch JM, Weeks T, Giles R et al. N Eng J Med 1990;322:1836–1841.
25. Sollid SJ, Markussen G, Gjede H et al. J Exp Med 1989;169:345–350.
26. Scharf SJ, Freidman A, Steinman L et al. Proc Natl Acad Sci USA 1989;86:6215–6219.
27. Nomura N, Ota M, Tsuji K et al. Tissue Antigens 1991;38:53–59.
28. Ota M, Seki T, Fukushima N et al. Tissue Antigens 1992;39:187–202.
29. Ota M, Seki T, Nomura N et al. Tissue Antigens. 1991;38:60–71
30. Kunkel HG, Ahrens JR, Eisenmenger WJ et al. J Clin Invest 1951;30:654.
31. Soloway RD, Summerskill WHJ, Baggenstoss AH et al. Gastroenterology 1972;63:358–365.
32. Ohta Y. Gastroenterologia Jpn 1993;28(suppl 4):128–133.
33. Nakanuma Y, Harada K, Nonomura A et al. In: Nishioka M, Toda G, Zeniya M (eds) Autoimmune Hepatitis, Amsterdam: Elsevier Science, 1994;85–127.
34. Mackay IR, Taft LI, Cowling DC. Lancet 1956;2:1323–1326.
35. Tan EM. Adv Immunol 1989;44:93–151
36. Toda G, Zeniya M, Aizawa Y et al. In: Nishioka M, Toda G, Zeniya M (eds) Autoimmune Hepatitis, Amsterdam: Elsevier Science, 1994;55–67.
37. Konikoff F, Isenberg DA, Barrison I. Hepatogastroenterol 1989;36:341–345.
38. Wood JR, Czaja AJ, Beaver SJ et al. Hepatology 1986;6:976–980.
39. Mackay IR. In: Krawitt EL, Wiesner RH (eds) Autoimmune Liver Diseases, New York: Raven Press, 1991;21–42.
40. Zeniya M, Aizawa Y, Watanabe F et al. Liver 1994;14:206–212.
41. Tsuji T, Sakaguchi K. In: Tsuji T, Yamada G (eds) Immune Response and Interferon Treatment in Viral Hepatitis, Tokyo: Nankodo, 1992;54–57.
42. Vogel W, Penner E. In: Krawitt EL, Wiesner RH (eds) Autoimmune Liver Diseases, New York: Raven Press, 1991;111–122.
43. Smeenk R, van der Lelij G, Swaak T. Arthritis Rheum 1982;25:631–638.
44. Gurian LE, Rogoff TM, Ware AJ et al. Hepatology 1985;5:397–402.
45. Tan EM, Feltkamp TEW, Alarcon-Segovia D. Arthritis Rheuma 1988;31:128–131.
46. Terada S, Morshed SA, Nishioka M. In: Nishioka M, Toda G, Zeniya M (eds) Autoimmune Hepatitis, Amsterdam: Elsevier Science, 1984;177–184.
47. Whittingham SF, Irwin J, Mackay IR et al. Gastroenterology 1966;51:499–505.
48. Czaja AJ. In: Czaja AJ, Dickson ER (eds) Chronic Active Hepatitis. The Mayo Clinic Experience, New York: Marcel Dekker, 1986;105–126.
49. Maddrey WC. Hepatology 1987;7:1372–1375.
50. Czaja AJ. Ann Intern Med 1993;119:510–515.
51. Odievre AM, Maggiore G, Homberg J-C. Hepatology 1983;3:407–409.
52. Manns M, Gerken G, Kyriatsoulis A. Lancet 1987;i:292–294.
53. Manns MP. In: Nishioka M, Toda G, Zeniya M (eds) Autoimmune Hepatitis, Amsterdam: Elsevier Science, 1994;165–175.

54. Homberg JC, Abuaf N, Bernard Q. et al. Hepatology 1991;1:1333–1339.
55. Michel G, Ritter A, Gerken G et al. Lancet1992;339:267–269.
56. Czaja AJ, Manns MP, Homburger HA. Gastroenterology 1992;103:1290–1293.
57. Garson JA, Lenzi M, Ring C et al. J Med Virol 1991;34:223–225.
58. Lenzi M, Ballardini G, Fusconi M et al. Lancet 1990;335:258–260.
59. Lunel F, Abuaf N, Frangeul L et al. Hepatology 1992;16:630–636.
60. Manns MP, Griffin KJ, Sullivan KF et al. J Clin Inves 1991;88:1370–1378.
61. Manns MP. Semin Liver Dis 1991;11:205–214.
62. Czaja AJ, Carpenter HA, Manns MP. Gastroenterology 1993;105:1522–1526.
63. McFarlane IG. Clin Sci 1983;64:127–135.
64. Schwartz AL. CRC Crit Rev Biochem 1984;16:207–233.
65. Tolleshaug H, Berg T, Nilsson M et al. Biochim Biophys Acta 1977;499:73–84.
66. Hubbard AL, Wilson G, Ashwell G et al. J Cell Biol 1979;83:47–64.
67. McFarlane MB, McSorley CG, Vergani D et al. J Hepatol 1986;3:196–205.
68. Poralla T, Treichel U, Lohr H et al. Sem Liver Dis 1991;11:215–222.
69. Treichel U, Poralla T, Hess G et al. Hepatology 1990;11:606–612.
70. McFarlane MB, McFarlane IG. In: Nishioka M, Toda G, Zeniya M (eds) Autoimmune Hepatitis, Amsterdam: Elsevier Science, 1994;143–164.
71. Toda G, Ikeda Y, Hashimoto N et al. Clin Exp Immunol 1983;54:661–670.
72. Toda G, Ikeda Y, Kashiwagi M et al. Hepatology 1990;12:671–675.
73. Toda G, Zeniya M. Int Med 1993;32:913–916.
74. Laitinen O, Vhheri A. Lancet 1974;1:194–195.
75. Trigger DR. Ann Clin Res 1976;8:174–180.
76. Haukenes G, Matre R, Tonder O et al. J Hepatol 1990;11:389.
77. Robertson DAF, Zhang SL, Guy EC. Lancet 1987;2:9–11.
78. Kalland K-H, Endresen C, Haukennes G et al. Lancet1989;1:1390.
79. Bulkey BH, Heizer WD, Goldfinger SE et al. Lancet 1970;2:1323–1324.
80. Shulman NR, Hirschman RJ, Barker LF. Ann Intern Med 1970;72:257–261.
81. Soloway RD, Summerskill WHJ, Baggenstoss AH et al. Gastroenterology, 1972;65:820–826.
82. Esteban JI, Esteban R, Viladomiu L et al. Lancet 1989;2:294–297.
83. Kuo G, Choo QL, Alter HJ. Science 1989;244:362–364.
84. Lenzi M, Johnson PJ, McFarlane IG et al. Lancet 1991;338:227–280.
85. Onji M, Nonaka T, Horiike N et al. Gastroenterologia Jpn 1993;28(suppl 4):134–138.
86. McFarlane IG, Smith HM, Johnson PJ et al. Lancet,1990;335:754–757.
87. Ikeda Y, Toda G, Hashimoto N et al. Lancet 1990;335:1345–1346.
88. Soloway RD, Summerskill WHJ, Baggenstoss AH et al. Gastroenterology 1972;63:820–826.
89. Czaja AJ. Gastroenterology clinics of North America 1994;23:547–566.
90. Choi Y, Kotzin B, Herron L et al. Proc Natl Acad Sci USA 1989;86:8941–8945.
91. Tomonaga B, Mak TW. Ann Rev Immunol 1987;5:585–620.
92. Sumida T, Yonaha F, Maeda T et al. J Clin Invest 1992;89:681–685.

Progress in Hepatology Vol. 1.
Cellular and Molecular Biology.
M. Yamanaka, K. Okabe and G. Toda, editors.

Risk factors for development of alcoholic liver cirrhosis

Masayoshi Yamauchi[1], Yoshihiko Maezawa[1], Mitsuru Ohata[1], Hisato Nakajima[1], Mitsuhiro Ichikawa[2], Gotaro Toda[1]

[1]First Department of Internal Medicine, The Jikei University School of Medicine, Tokyo, Japan; and [2]Tokyo Medical Center of Alcohol Related Disability, Tokyo, Japan

Abstract. Alcoholic liver cirrhosis is found in only a subpopulation of alcoholic patients. Risk factors for development of alcoholic liver cirrhosis might be explained by a number of mechanisms including difference in ethanol metabolism, nutrition such as low-protein and high-fat diet, especially vegetable oil, sex difference, and genetic factors. Genetic polymorphisms have been reported in alcohol dehydrogenase 2 (ADH2), aldehyde dehydrogenase 2 (ALDH2), 5′-flanking region of P450IIEI, and pro α 2(I) collagen genes. This article reviews the genetic factors for development of alcoholism and alcoholic liver cirrhosis. The alcoholics had significantly higher frequencies of the $ADH2^1$ and $ALDH2^1$ alleles than did the healthy subjects. Among the alcoholics, the frequency of the $ADH2^2$ and *c1* allele of the P450IIE1 was significantly higher in cirrhotic than in noncirrhotic alcoholic patients. A specific haplotype pattern of the pro α (I) collagen gene with homozygous for the presence of *EcoR* I and heterozygous for *MsP* I polymorphisms was found more frequently in patients with liver cirrhosis than those with noncirrhotic alcoholic liver disease. The screening for the genetic polymorphisms of alcohol-metabolizing enzymes and the specific haplotype of pro α (I) collagen gene may identify those alcoholics at increased risk of developing liver cirrhosis.

Chronic ethanol consumption has been associated with alcoholic liver disease. However, alcoholic liver cirrhosis develops in only a subpopulation of alcoholic patients [1]. A number of studies have looked for differences in ethanol metabolism [2,3], nutrition [3–7], sex difference [8,9], hepatitis C virus (HCV) [10], and certain human lymphocyte antigen (HLA) types [11–13] to explain susceptibility to alcoholic liver cirrhosis (Table 1). Genetic polymorphisms have been reported in alcohol dehydrogenase 2 (ADH2), aldehyde dehydrogenase 2 (ALDH2), 5′-flanking region of P450IIEI, and pro α 2(I) collagen genes [12–18]. Recently, several studies on the association between the polymorphisms and alcoholic liver cirrhosis have been reported [18–28]. In this manuscript, we demonstrate the risk factors for the development of alcoholic liver cirrhosis.

Address for correspondence: Masayoshi Yamauchi, M.D., First Department of Internal Medicine, The Jikei University School of Medicine, 3-25-8, Nishi-shinbashi, Minato-ku, Tokyo 105, Japan. Phone: (03)3433-1111. Fax: (03)3435-0569.

Table 1. Risk factors for development of alcoholic liver cirrhosis

1. Nutritional factors
Low protein, high fat, polyunsaturated fat
2. Sex
Female
3. Genetic polymorphisms of alcohol metabolizing enzymes
Alcohol dehydrogenase
Aldehyde dehydrogenase
P450IIE1
4. HLA types
5. Haplotype of type I collagen gene
6. Hepatitis C virus

Role of dietary factors

The hepatotoxicity of ethanol has been established by the demonstration that in the absence of dietary deficiencies, and even in the presence of protein-, vitamin-, and mineral-enriched diets, ethanol produces fatty liver with striking ultrastructural lesions, and fibrosis with cirrhosis in nonhuman primates [4]. However, alcoholic liver cirrhosis develops in only a subpopulation of alcohol-fed baboons [4] and human alcoholics [1]. By contrast, rats fed an ethanol-corn oil diet developed all of the features of alcoholic liver injury, whereas animals fed ethanol with saturated fat developed little or no hepatic damage in the Tsukamoto-French intragastric feeding model [6]. Recently it is emphasized that dietary fat, especially vegetable fat, is the most important factor for the development of alcoholic hepatic fibrosis [3,6,7,29]. Low-protein and high-fat diets are also important factors in the occurrence and progression of alcoholic liver disease [3,29].

We compared the differences in the nutritional background of the patients with alcoholic liver diseases between the USA and Japan. Alcohol contributed about 50% of total calorie intake in all or both sets of patients with alcoholic liver cirrhosis [30]. American patients with alcoholic liver cirrhosis had significantly higher fat intake than Japanese patients as shown in Table 2 ($p < 0.001$). Protein intake was 8.9 Cal% of total calorie intake of both patients. Laboratory data such as serum levels of bilirubin and albumin showed more abnormal values in American patients than in Japanese. These results suggest that dietary fat may be involved in the clinical differences in the severity of alcoholic liver disease, which exist between American and Japanese patients. To clarify the role of the amount of protein and fat in the development of alcoholic hepatic fibrosis, male Wistar rats were paired fed isocalorically with standard diet (15 Cal% of protein, 15 Cal% of fat), low-protein diet (5 Cal% of protein, 15 Cal% of fat), and low-protein + high-fat diet (5 Cal% of protein, 35 Cal% of fat) with or without 36 Cal% of

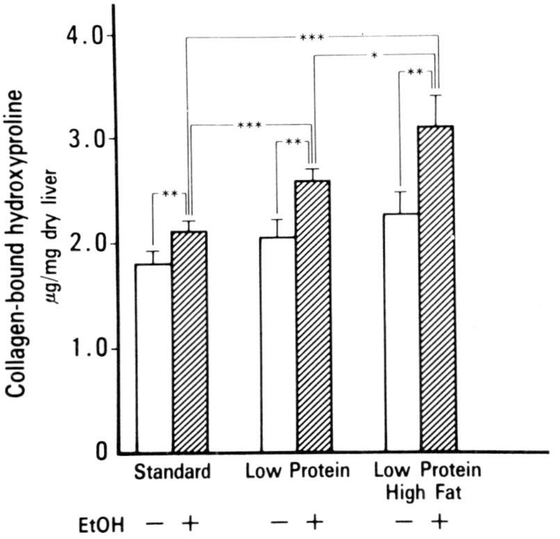

Fig. 1. Effect of chronic ethanol consumption on hepatic collagen-bound hydroxyproline in low-protein- and/or high-fat-fed rats. *, $p<0.10$; **, $p<0.05$; ***, $p<0.01$; ****, $p<0.001$.

Table 2. Dietary background in the patients with alcoholic liver cirrhosis between USA and Japan

	USA	Japan
Total calories/BEE[a]	1.88 ± 0.14	1.78 ± 0.11
Alcohol calories/BEE	0.98 ± 0.11	0.87 ± 0.11
Nonalcohol calories/BEE	0.93 ± 0.08	0.91 ± 0.07
Protein calories/BEE	0.17 ± 0.01	0.17 ± 0.02
Fat calories/BEE	0.39 ± 0.04	0.18 ± 0.02[b]
Carbohydrate calories/BEE	0.40 ± 0.06	0.53 ± 0.05

All values are expressed as mean ± S.E.
[a]Basal energy expenditure. Male: 66+ (13.7 × weight) + (5 × height) − (6.8 × age); female 655+ (9.6 × weight) + (1.7 × height) − (4.7 × age). [b]$p<0.001$ vs. USA.

ethanol for 12 weeks. Hepatic collagen-bound hydroxyproline was much higher in the low-protein + high-fat–ethanol group compared to the low-protein–ethanol and the standard–ethanol groups (Fig. 1) [3,31].

We also determined the effect of unsaturated and saturated fat on the development of alcoholic liver disease [7,32]. According to the nutritional backgrounds of American patients with alcoholic liver cirrhosis [30], male Sprague-Dawley rats were paired fed isocalorically with safflower oil and beef fat (8 Cal% of protein, 20 Cal% of fat) with or without 46 Cal% of ethanol for 8 weeks. Serum glutamate pyruvate transaminase activity as well as hepatic collagen-bound hydroxyproline was much higher in the safflower–

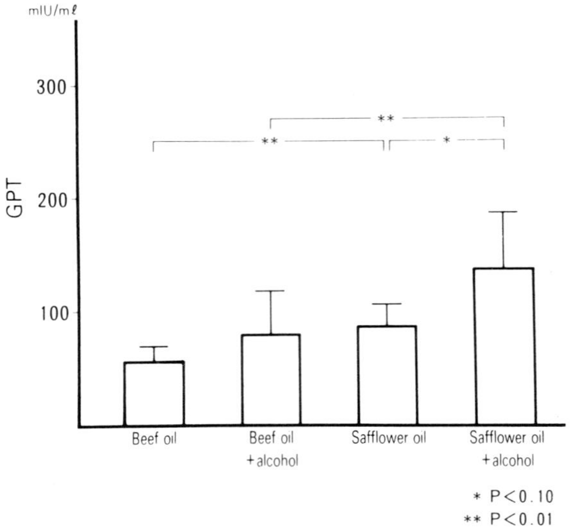

Fig. 2. Effect of chronic ethanol consumption on plasma GPT activity in beef or safflower oil-fed rats. *, $p<0.10$; **, $p<0.05$; ***, $p<0.01$; ****, $p<0.005$.

ethanol group compared to the beef–ethanol group (Fig. 2) [7]. These data show that dietary fat is the important factor, not only quantitatively but also qualitatively, for the development of alcoholic liver cirrhosis. Nanji et al. [6] have reported the degree of histopathological abnormality correlated with the linoleic acid content of fat in the diet (tallow 0.7%, lard 2.5%, corn oil 56.6%). They also have postulated that linoleic acid facilitates the development of alcoholic hepatic fibrosis. Precise mechanisms underlying this linoleic acid effect are unknown, but the following hypotheses have been offered [33]: (a) enhanced susceptibility to lipid peroxidation caused by increased intake of polyunsaturated fat [34]; (b) induction of the microsomal P450IIE1 by polyunsaturated fat [35,36] and subsequent enhancement of lipid peroxidation by P450IIE1-derived free radicals [37]; (c) aggravation of centrilobular liver hypoxia by induction of a microsomal ethanol oxidizing system (MEOS) that uses more oxygen than alcohol dehydrogenase in the oxidation of ethanol; (d) activation of macrophages or Kupfer cells by unsaturated fatty acids [38,39]; and (e) sensitization of Ito cells by increased intake of polyunsaturated fat [40].

Effect of sex

The average cirrhogenic dose of alcohol as well as the threshold amount is lower in women than in men. The incidence of chronic advanced liver disease

Table 3. Effect of chronic ethanol consumption on ethanol elimination rate between male and female rats

		μmol/ml/hr	mM/kg.body weight/hr
Female	Control	12.32 ± 1.43[a,c]	8.06 ± 0.88[b]
	Alcohol	9.19 ± 1.06	7.41 ± 0.55
Male	Control	9.13 ± 0.67	6.66 ± 0.30[d]
	Alcohol	9.76 ± 0.61	7.83 ± 0.82

[a]$p < 0.005$ vs. Male Control; [b]$p < 0.025$ vs. Male Control; [c]$p < 0.01$ vs. Female Alcohol; [d]$p < 0.05$ vs. Male Alcohol.

is higher among women than among men for those with similar histories of alcohol abuse [8,9]. Sex differences in ethanol metabolism have been reported for the liver [41,42] and for the stomach [43,44]. Hepatic alcohol dehydrogenase (ADH) activity is suppressed by testosterone and its derivatives, both in vivo [45] and in vitro [46]. In our experimental animals, it was observed that rates of ethanol metabolism decreased significantly in the ethanol-fed female rats, associated with a decrease in hepatic ADH activity, where no such effect was found in male rats (Table 3) [47]. We also found sex difference in liver regeneration and ornithine decarboxylase (ODC) protein after acute ethanol administration to hepatectomized rats. Liver weight, total protein contents and DNA synthesis were significantly decreased in the female ethanol group accompanied with a significant decrease in ODC protein (Fig. 3) [48]. These data indicate that the inhibitory effect of liver regenera-

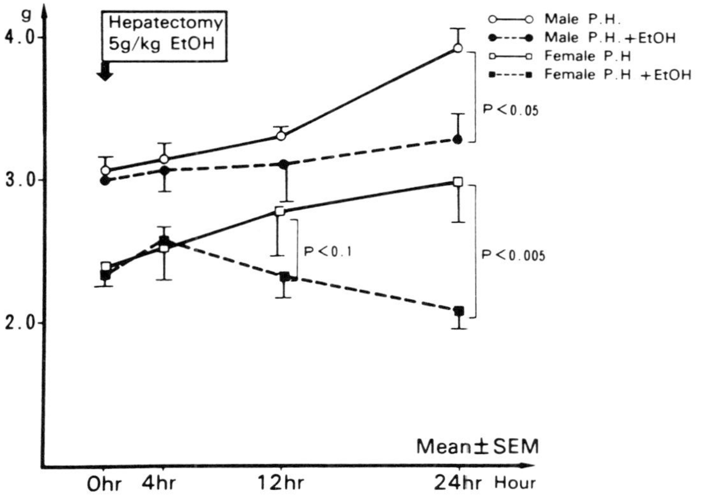

Fig. 3. Effect of acute ethanol administration (5 g/kg) and partial hepatectomy on the weight of regenerating rat livers.

tion by alcohol is more prominent in females, which may be one reason why females are more susceptible to developing liver cirrhosis than males.

Women also have lower gastric ADH activity than men [43], at least below the age of 50 years [44]. This decrease in ADH activity may contribute to the reduced first-pass metabolism of ethanol and associated raised ethanol blood concentrations. The higher blood ethanol level, in turn, also may contribute to the greater susceptibility of women to alcohol.

Polymorphisms of alcohol-metabolizing enzyme genes

Alcohol and aldehyde dehydrogenase genotypes and alcoholism in Japanese men

We studied 96 male Japanese alcoholics, aged 32 to 72 (average age 52.1 ± 1.0), who had consumed more than 120 g of ethanol daily for at least 10 years. Alcohol dependence was diagnosed on the basis of DSM-III-R criteria [49] by two psychiatrists. The mean cumulative alcohol consumption of these men was $1{,}266.5 \pm 80.8$ kg of ethanol. Sixty nonrelated healthy Japanese men were also studied. The genotypes of the *ADH2* and *ALDH2* loci were determined, using leukocyte DNA by the restriction fragment length polymorphism by polymerase chain reaction [50,51]. The frequency of the three *ADH2* genotypes in the 60 healthy subjects in this study was similar to that previously reported for the Japanese population [52]. The frequency of the genotype $ADH2^1/ADH2^1$ was significantly higher in the alcoholics than in the healthy subjects ($p < 0.001$, $\chi^2 = 17.921$) (Table 4) [53]. The frequency of the $ADH2^1$ allele was 0.458 in the alcoholics, and 0.217 in the healthy subjects. Thus, the $ADH2^1$ allele was found more frequently in the alcoholics than in the healthy subjects ($p < 0.001$, $\chi^2 = 17.572$). The $ALDH2^1$ allele frequency was also significantly higher in the alcoholics than in the healthy subjects (Table 4) [53]. In the latter group, it was almost the same as that previously reported [25,54] ($p < 0.001$, $\chi^2 = 12.894$).

The $\beta 2 \beta 2$ isozyme encoded by $ADH2^2$ has a 40-fold higher V_{max} than does the $\beta 1 \beta 1$ isozyme encoded by $ADH2^1$ [2]. Under predicted physiologic conditions, the specific activity of $\beta 2 \beta 2$ enzyme was 80× higher than that of the $\beta 1 \beta 1$ enzymes [55,56]. In other words, $\beta 2 \beta 2$ enzymes generate larger amounts of acetaldehyde than do $\beta 1 \beta 1$ enzymes. More acetaldehyde is generated by the alcoholics with the $ADH2^2$ allele than by those with the $ADH2^1$ allele. In the homozygote of the mutant *ALDH2* gene, acetaldehyde metabolism in the liver was severely impaired because of the absence of hepatic *ALDH2* activity [57]. These data suggest that alcoholics are less likely to have enyzmes that cause the accumulation of acetaldehyde, a situation associated with unpleasant symptoms most commonly described in the

Table 4. Genotype and allele frequency of ADH2 and ALDH2 genes in alcoholics and healthy subjects

	ADH2 genotype			2^1 allele frequency	ALDH genotype			2^1 allele frequency
	ADH2^1/2^1	ADH2^1/2^2	ADH2^2/2^2	ADH2^1	ALDH2^1/2^1	ALDH2^1/2^2	ALDH2^2/2^2	ALDH2^1
Alcoholics	30(31.2%)[a]	28(29.2%)	38(39.6%)	0.458[b]	76(79.2%)[a]	20(20.8%)	0(0%)	0.896[b]
Healthy subjects	2(3.3%)	22(36.7%)	36(60.0%)	0.217	34(56.7%)	20(33.3%)	6(10.0%)	0.733

[a]$p<0.001$ vs. Healthy subjects; [b]$p<0.001$ vs. Healthy subjects.

Table 5. Genotype and allele frequency of ADH2 gene in alcoholics depending on alcohol-drinking pattern

	ADH2 genotype			Gene frequency	
	ADH2^1/2^1	ADH2^1/2^2	ADH2^2/2^2	ADH2^1	ADH2^2
Intermittent drinking	6(24.0%)	6(24.0%)	13(52.0%)	18(36.0%)	32(64.0%)[a,b]
Mixed type	4(50.0%)	1(12.5%)	3(37.5%)	9(56.3%)	7(43.7%)
Continuous drinking	19(40.4%)	13(27.7%)	15(31.9%)	51(54.3%)	43(45.7%)

[a]$p<0.10$ vs. Continuous drinking type; [b]$p<0.05$ vs. Mixed type + Continuous drinking type.

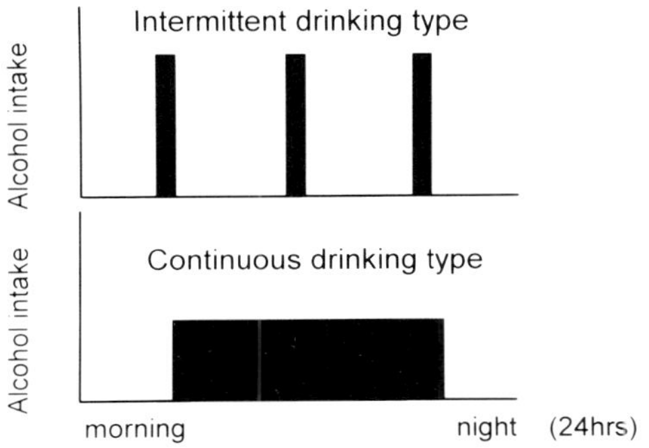

Fig. 4. Alcohol drinking pattern.

flushing syndrome of *ALDH2* deficiency which makes alcohol consumption uncomfortable.

We classified the alcoholics into three groups according to their drinking pattern as shown on Fig. 4, namely intermittent drinking type, continuous drinking type and mixed type. As shown in Table 5, in the alcoholics, the *ADH2*^{2} allele frequency is higher in the intermittent drinking type than in the

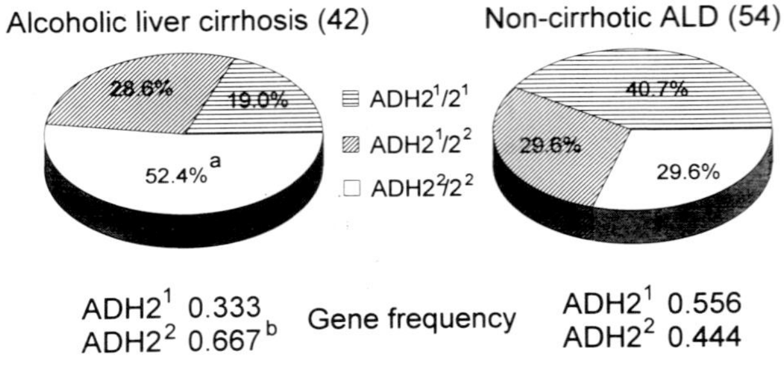

Fig. 5. Genotype and allele frequency of ADH2 in patients with alcoholic liver disease. [a], $p < 0.05$ vs noncirrhotic alcoholic liver disease; [b], $p < 0.01$ vs noncirrhotic alcoholic liver disease.

continuous drinking type. These data suggest that those with the $ALDH2^2/ALDH2^2$ genotype cannot develop alcoholism. By contrast, those who have either the $ADH2^2$ or $ADH2^1$ allele could develop alcoholism, although their alcohol-drinking pattern is different.

Genetic polymorphisms of alcohol-metabolizing enzymes and alcoholic liver cirrhosis in Japanese men

Alcohol dehydrogenase 2 genotypes and alcoholic liver cirrhosis

Fifty-four patients had noncirrhotic liver disease, including normal liver function, fatty liver, nonspecific reaction and hepatic fibrosis. The 42 patients with cirrhotic liver disease all had alcoholic liver cirrhosis. The frequency of the genotype $ADH2^2/ADH2^2$ was significantly higher in cirrhotic than in noncirrhotic alcoholic patients ($p < 0.05$, Fig. 5) [24]. While the frequency of the $ADH2^2$ allele was 0.444 in the noncirrhotic group, it was 0.667 in the cirrhotic group. Thus, the $ADH2^2$ allele was present more frequently in cirrhotic than in noncirrhotic patients ($p < 0.01$, Fig. 5).

The involvement of polymorphic ADH2 genes in alcoholic cirrhosis has been reported in previous studies [20–24,28]. The association between the ADH2 polymorphisms and alcoholic cirrhosis is summarized in Table 6. A study from western France by Couzigou et al. [20] has shown no differences in *ADH2* or *ADH3* allele frequencies between patients with cirrhosis and controls. Day et al. [21], however, have identified an association between *ADH3* genotypes and cirrhosis in a population from northeast England. Recently Sherman et al. [22] have reported an association of a restriction fragment length polymorphism (RFLP) on Southern hybridization with a 1.3 Kb genomic DNA probe to the *ADH2* gene with alcoholic-induced liver damage in a population from the UK. These results remain inconclusive. In European or White American populations, the $\beta 1$ isoform, encoded by

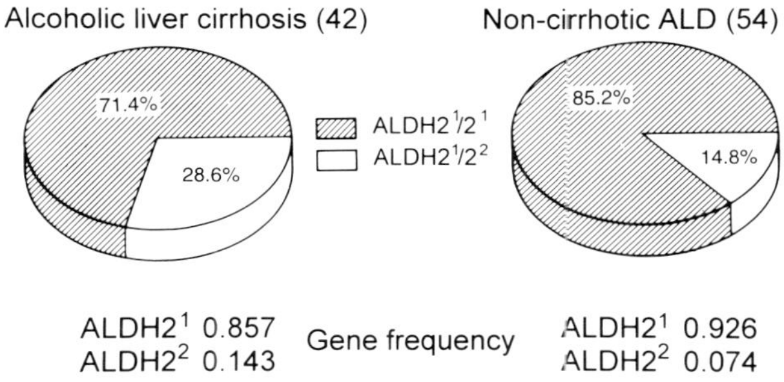

Fig. 6. Genotype and allele frequency of ALDH2 in patients with alcoholic liver disease.

Table 6. Gene frequency of ADH2 gene in patients with alcoholic liver cirrhosis

	Alcoholic cirrhosis	Noncirrhotic ALD[a]	Healthy subjects
Couzigou et al (1990)	ADH2^1/2^2:0.978/0.022(46)[b]	–	0.987/0.013(39)
Day et al (1993)	ADH2^1/2^2:1.000/0 (59)	1.000/0 (13)	0.994/0.006(79)
Sherman et al (1993)	A/B :0.268/0.732(28)	0.750/0.250(4)	0.850/0.150(23)
Tanaka et al (1993)	ADH2^1/2^2:0.450/0.550(30)	0.364/0.636(33)	0.250/0.750(30)[c]
Chao et al (1994)	ADH2^1/2^2:0.430/0.570(27)	0.520/0.480(37)	0.270/0.730(47)
Yamauchi et al (1994)	ADH2^1/2^2:0.304/0.696(46)	0.574/0.426(34)	0.217/0.783(60)

[a]Alcoholic liver disease; [b]number of cases; [c]nonalcoholic liver disease

ADH2^1, is most common, while the β 2 isoform, encoded by the *ADH2*^{2} allele, is predominant in Asian populations. A study on the association between *ADH2* polymorphism and alcoholic liver cirrhosis should be performed in Orientals.

Aldehyde dehydrogenase 2 genotypes and alcoholic liver cirrhosis

The genotype and allele frequencies of *ALDH2* were not different between the noncirrhotic and the cirrhotic groups (Fig. 6). However, mean cumulative alcohol intake was significantly lower in the cirrhotic patients with *ALDH2* heterozygotes than in those with *ALDH2*^{1}/*ALDH2*^{1} genotype, which was the same as that reported previously [25]. The *ALDH2* gene may also be a determinant in the development of alcoholic cirrhosis.

P450IIE1 genotypes and alcoholic liver cirrhosis

The functional properties of cytochrome P450IIE1, an ethanol-inducible isozyme of liver microsomal P-450, suggest that this enzyme plays an important role in ethanol metabolism [58]. Genetic polymorphisms in the 5′-flanking region of the human cytochrome P450IIE1 gene have recently

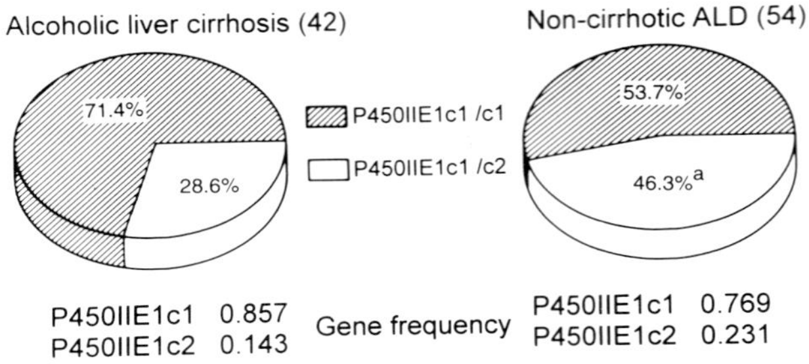

Fig. 7. Genotype and allele frequency of P450IIE1 in patients with alcoholic liver disease. [a], $p < 0.10$ vs alcoholic liver cirrhosis.

been reported [17]. The frequencies of two RFLPs, c1 (*Rsa*I site +, *Pst*I site −) and c2 (*Rsa*I site −, *Pst*I site +), were found to be 0.80 and 0.20, respectively, in unrelated Japanese individuals [17,26]. Figure 7 shows the frequency of each P450IIE1 RFLP in the cirrhotic and noncirrhotic groups. The frequency of the type B, c1/c2 heterozygote, RFLPs was higher in non-cirrhotic than in cirrhotic patients [26]. Ingelman-Sundberg et al. [27] have reported that allele frequencies of the P450IIE1 are 0.96 for c1 allele and 0.04 for c2 in 114 Italian healthy subjects. The frequency of c2 allele is significantly higher in our Japanese subjects than in the Italian population ($p < 0.001$, $\chi^2 = 16.684$). He also has reported that no difference in c1 allele frequency was observed between the patients with alcoholic liver cirrhosis and healthy controls. Due to the relatively low frequency of the rare c2 allele, the difference in the distribution must be verified using a larger group of Caucasian individuals.

Ethanol metabolism and schematic representation of its link to liver cirrhosis

Figure 8 shows the association between alcohol metabolism and the schematic representation of its link to liver cirrhosis. Beta 1 encoded $ADH2^1$ is the most common in European or White American populations, while about 65–85% of Japanese and Chinese have isoenzymes with β 2 subunits, encoded by the $ADH2^2$ allele [16,55]. The $\beta 2 \beta 2$ enzyme is approximately 20× more active in ethanol oxidation than $\beta 1 \beta 1$ [55], so that $\beta 2 \beta 2$ generates more acetaldehyde and the reduced form of nicotinamide adenine dinucleotide (NADH) than $\beta 1 \beta 1$. ADH-mediated oxidation of ethanol to acetaldehyde also generates NADH, which in turn reduces pyruvate to lactate [59]. Lactate has been shown to stimulate fibrogenesis of the liver [60]. Hayashi et al. [17] have reported that chloramphenicol acetyltransferase (CAT) activity is 10× higher in Hep G2 cells with type C (c2/c2) P450IIE1 alleles than in cells with type A (c1/c1) alleles. The transcriptional activity may be higher in type B patients than in type A. Since P450IIE1-catalyzed ethanol oxidation results in

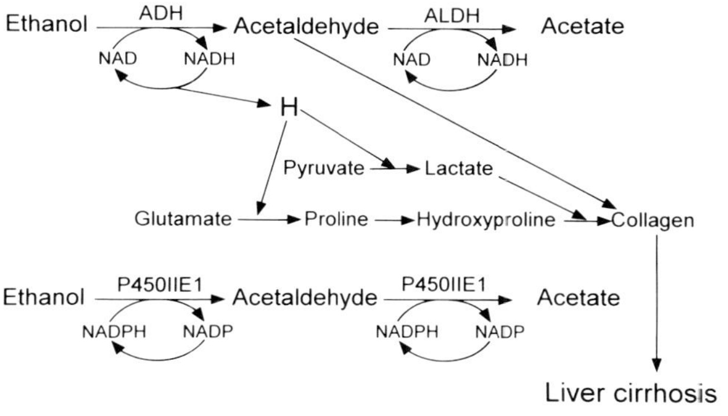

Fig. 8. Ethanol metabolism and schematic representation of its link to liver cirrhosis.

the formation of acetaldehydes and free radicals capable of peroxidizing cell membranes, enhanced P450IIE1 concentrations in liver microsomes after chronic ethanol intake may contribute to the development of alcoholic cirrhosis [37,61,62]. Our finding that alcoholics with the c1 allele are more susceptible to alcoholic cirrhosis is the opposite of what one might expect. However, P450IIE1 can oxidize ethanol to acetaldehyde without producing NADH. This may be one reason why alcoholics with the c1 allele are more susceptible to alcoholic cirrhosis. Recently, opposite results regarding the association between the P450IIE1 polymorphisms and alcoholic cirrhosis in England have been reported [63].

Haplotype of pro α (I) collagen gene and alcoholic liver cirrhosis (COL1A2)

A significant association of a particular RFLP haplotype of the COL1A2 locus and alcoholic cirrhosis has been reported by some investigators [18,19], but not confirmed by others [64]. In our study, the frequency of the haplotype with polymorphic sites of EcoRI (+, +) and MspI (+, −) is significantly higher in the patients with alcoholic liver cirrhosis than in those with noncirrhotic alcoholic liver disease ($p<0.05$) (Fig. 9) [19]. Weiner et al. [18] also investigated the haplotype analysis of the type I collagen gene and its association with alcoholic liver cirrhosis in humans. They concluded that patients with a heterozygous pattern for the presence of the *EcoR* I polymorphism and a homozygous pattern for the presence of the *Msp* I polymorphism are susceptible for developing cirrhosis. But our data are different from Weiner's results. The reason for this discrepancy may be due to the different ethnic backgrounds of the patients studied. The patients they studied were of various races. In our study, the patients were all Japanese, a single race. Japan has a stable population, providing an ideal homogeneous

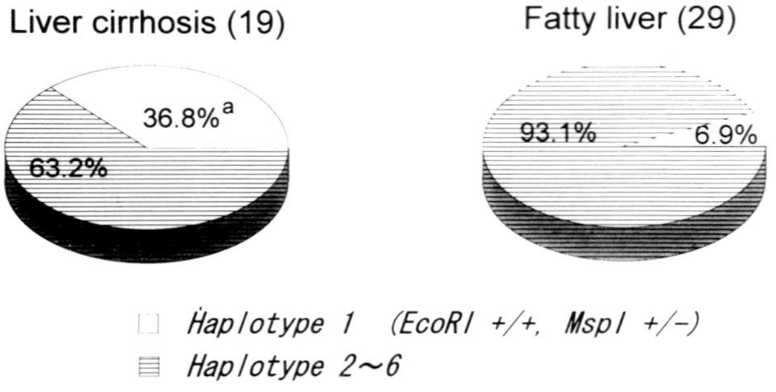

Fig. 9. Frequency of haplotype of Pro α (I) Collagen Gene between patients with alcoholic liver cirrhosis and fatty liver. [a], $p<0.05$ vs fatty liver.

group in which to undertake genetic studies. In fact, Monica et al. [65] have reported that two pro α 2(I) collagen gene RFLPs were more polymorphic in an Italian population than in an English Caucasian population.

References

1. Marbet UA, Bianchi L, Meury U et al. J Hepatol 1987;4:364–372.
2. Bosron WF, Li TK. Hepatology 1986;6:502–510.
3. Kimura K, Yamauchi M, Fujisawa K. In: Kuriyaa K, Takada A, Ishii H (eds) Biomedical and Social Aspects of Alcohol and Alcoholism. Amsterdam: Elsevier Science BV, 1988.
4. Lieber CS, Jones DP, Leonore MD. J Clin Invest 1965;44:1009–1021.
5. Best CH, Hartroft WS, Lucas CC et al. Br Med J 1949;2:1001–1006.
6. Nanji AA, Mendenhal CL, French SW. Alcohol Cli Exp Re 1989;13:1–1.
7. Yamauchi M, Hirakawa J, Ohata M et al. Alcohol and Metabolism 1992;11:86–91.
8. Morgan M, Sherlock S. Br Med J 1977;1:939–941.
9. Pequignot G, Chabert C, Eydoux H et al. Revue Alcoholism 1974;20:191–202.
10. Fong T-L, Kanel GC, Conrad A et al. Hepatology 1994;19:554–557.
11. Saunder JB, Hainer A, Portman B et al. Lancet 1982;19:1381–1384.
12. Faizallah R, Woodrow JC, Krasner NK et al. BMJ 1982;285:533–534.
13. Monteiro E, Alves MP, Quintas I et al. Hepatology 1984;4:1047.
14. Smith M. Adv Hum Genet 1986;15:249–290.
15. Yoshida A, Hsu LC, Yasunami M. Prog Nucleic Acid Res Mol Biol 1991;40:255–287.
16. Goedde HW, Agarwal DP, Fritze G et al. Hum Genet 1992;88:344–346.
17. Hayashi S-I, Watanabe J, Kawajiri K. J Biochem 1991;110:559–565.
18. Weiner FR, Eskreis DS, Compton KV et al. Molec Aspects Med 1988;10:159–168.
19. Ohata M. Jikeikai Med J 1933;40:401–412.
20. Couzigou P, Fleury B, Groppi A et al. Alcohol and Alcoholism 1990;25:623–626.
21. Day CP, Bashir R, James OFW et al. Hepatology 1991;14:798–801.
22. Sherman DI, Ward RJ, Warren-Perry M et al. Br Med J 1993;307:1388–1390.
23. Chao YC, Liou SR, Chung YY et al. Hepatology 1994;19:360–366.
24. Yamauchi M, Maezawa Y, Mizuhara Y et al. Hepatology Polymorphisms in alchohol metabolizing genes and alchoholic cirrhosis in Japanese patients: A multivariate analysis (in press).

25. Enomoto N, Takase S, Takada N et al. Hepatology 1991;13:1071–1075.
26. Maezawa Y, Yamauchi M, Toda G. Am J Gastroenterol 1994;89:561–565.
27. Ingelman-Sundberg M, Johansson I, Yin H et al. Alcohol 1993;10:447–452.
28. Tanaka F, Omata M, Tsukada E et al. Nippon Rinshou 1993;51:400–406.
29. Tsukamot H, Towner SJ, Ciofalo LM et al. Hepatology 1986;6:814–822.
30. Yamauchi M, Kimura K, Fujisawa K et al. Acta Hepatol Jap 1989;30:173–177.
31. Kimura K. Tokyo Jikeikai Medical J 1990;105:701–713.
32. Yamauchi M, Hirakawa J, Mizuhara Y et al. Jpn Clin Nutrition 1992;80:366–371.
33. Tsukamoto H, Gall K, French SW. Hepatology 1990;12:599–608.
34. Lokesh BR, Mathur SN, Spector AA. J Lipid Res 1981;22:905–915.
35. Marshall WJ, McLean AEM. Biochem J 1971;122:569–573.
36. Kanayama R, Takase S, Matsuda Y et al. Biochem Pharmacol 1984;33:3283–3287.
37. Castillo T, Koop DR, Kamimura S et al. Hepatology 1992;16:992–996.
38. Bromberg Y, Pick E. Cell Immunol 1983;79:240–252.
39. Nanji AA, Saadrzadeh SMH, Thomas P et al. Life Science 1994;55:611–620.
40. Matsuoka M, Zhang M, Tsukamoto H. Hepatology 1990;11:173–185.
41. Arthur MJP, Lee A, Wright R. Cli Sci 1984;67:397–401.
42. Yamauchi M, Potter JJ, Mezey E. Hepatology 1988;8:243–247.
43. Frezza M, Di Padova C, Pozzato G et al. N Eng J Med 1990;322:95–99.
44. Seitz HK, Egerer G, Simanowski UA et al. Gut 1993;34:1433–1437.
45. Teschke R, Wiese B. J Endocrinol Invest 1982;5:243–250.
46. Mezey E, Potter JJ, Diehl AM. Biochem Pharmacol 1980;35:335–339.
47. Yamauchi M, Hirakawa J, Kimura K et al. Acta Hepatol Jpn 1989;30:643–648.
48. Nakajima H, Yamauchi M, Hirakawa J et al. Acta Hepatol Jpn 1990;22:610–616.
49. The American Psychiatric Association: Diagnostic and Statistical Manual of Mental Disorders. Third edition – revised. Washington, DC, 1987.
50. Xu Y, Carr LG, Bosron WF et al. Genomics 1988;2:209–214.
51. Harada S, Zhang S. Alcohol Alcoholism 1993;28(suppl 1A):11–13.
52. Ikuta T, Shibuya A, Yoshida A. Biochem Genet 1988;26:519–525.
53. Mezawa Y, Yamauchi M, Toda G et al. Alchohol metabolizing enzyme polymorphisms and alchoholism in Japan. Alcoolis Clin Exp Res (in press).
54. Shibuya A, Yoshida A. Am J Hum Genet 1988;43:744–748.
55. Bosron WF, Lumeng L, Li T-K. Molec Asp Med 1988;10:147–158.
56. Yoshida A, Impraim CC, Huang IY. J Biol Chem 256:12430–12436.
57. Takase S, Yasuhara M, Takada A et al. Alcohol 1990;7:37–41.
58. Lieber CS, DeCarli LM. J Biol Chem 1970;245:2505–2512.
59. Domschke S, Domschke W, Lieber CS. Life Sci 1974;15:1327–1334.
60. Savolainen ER, Leo MA, Timpl R et al. Gastroenterology 1984;87:777–787.
61. Koop DR, Crump BL, Nordblom GD et al. Proc Natl Acad Sci USA 1985;82:4065–4069.
62. Ryan DE, Koop DR, Thomas PE et al. Arch Biochem Biophys 1986;246:633–644.
63. Primohamed M, Quest LJ, Kitteringham NR et al. Hepatology 1994;20:317A.
64. Bashir R, Day CP, Jame OFW et al. J Hepatol 1992;16:316–319.
65. Monica M, Loredana C, Pier FP. Hum Genet 1989;83:369–372.

Progress in Hepatology Vol. 1.
Cellular and Molecular Biology.
M. Yamanaka, K. Okabe and G. Toda, editors.

Molecular pathogenesis of hepatocellular carcinoma in hepatitis B virus infection

Kazuhiko Koike, Kyoji Moriya, Hiroshi Yotsuyanagi, Yoshizumi Shintani, and Kiyoshi Kurokawa
First Department of Internal Medicine, University of Tokyo, Tokyo 113, Japan

Abstract. Hepatitis B virus HBx gene has been shown to induce hepatocellular carcinoma in transgenic mice and is implicated in hepatocarcinogenesis in human chronic hepatitis B virus infection. To further characterize the role of HBx gene in carcinogenesis, we first analyzed the preneoplastic liver in HBx-transgenic mice. From the age of 2 months, there appeared preneoplastic liver foci, which consisted of hepatocytes with vacuolations in their cytoplasm, but they did not progress until 12 months. Hepatocytes in these foci which showed relatively higher levels of HBx protein in cytoplasm than the surrounding tissues demonstrated increased DNA synthesis in their nuclei. We then established mouse fibroblast cell lines in which the expression of HBx gene is under the control of hormone-regulated promoter. Upon induction of the HBx gene, serum-depleted resting cells began to enter into the S-phase of the cell cycle. These results indicate that HBx gene has mitogenic activity both in vivo and in vitro and suggest that HBx gene may contribute to hepatocarcinogenesis by driving cells into deregulated cell cycle control. We propose a mechanism for hepatocarcinogenesis by which continued stimulation for cell cycle progression in vivo may lead to the development of hepatocellular carcinoma by placing hepatocytes in a subthreshold state for transformation.

Key words: cell cycle, HBx gene, NIH3T3 cells, transgenic mice.

Introduction

The association of hepatitis B virus (HBV) infection with the development of hepatocellular carcinoma (HCC) is well documented and has been the focus of research over the past twenty years [1,2]. The mechanism of hepatocarcinogenesis is, however, still unclear despite a number of studies on integrated HBV genomes and adjacent host sequences [3].

Recently, one of the four genes encoded by HBV, the HBx gene, has been found to be a viral transactivator [4]. Since then, a variety of genes have been shown to be activated by HBx protein. Activating a broad spectrum of genes, *HBx* gene is implicated in carcinogenesis as one of the causative factors [5].

Address for correspondence: Kazuhiko Koike, M.D., First Department of Internal Medicine, Faculty of Medicine, University of Tokyo, 7-3-1 Hongo, Bunkyo-ku, Tokyo 113, Japan. Phone +-81-3-3815-5411 ext 3004. Fax +-81-3-3812-5063.

We have shown previously, as an alternative mechanism, that the *HBx* gene could cause HCC using a transgenic mouse system [6]. In the present study, we first analyzed the events preceding the development of hepatic neoplasia in this transgenic system, and found that the *HBx* gene may play a role in hepatocarcinogenesis through its mitogenic activity. We then showed that *HBx* gene has a mitogenic activity in cultured cells as well, using an inducible gene expression system.

Materials and Methods

Transgenic mice

The production of the HBx transgenic mice has been reported [6]. Among 3 strains established, male mice of the H9 strain were used in the present study.

Immunohistochemistry

Tissue sections fixed in 10% neutral-buffered formalin or frozen sections were used for hematoxylin and eosin (H&E) staining or immunostaining. The *HBx* gene product in liver tissue was stained with a rabbit anti-HBx serum using an ABC kit (Vector Laboratories, Burlingame, CA, USA). Specificity control was carried out as described previously [7].

BrdU labeling

For bromo deoxyuridine (BrdU) incorporation studies, mice were given BrdU intraperitoneally, or cells were labeled in culture medium. After fixation, samples were stained with anti-BrdU antibody and visualized.

Flow cytometry

Flow cytometry was carried out on purified nuclear preparations. Nuclei were stained with propidium iodide and analyzed on a FACScan flow cytometer (Becton-Dickinson, San Jose, CA, USA).

Cell line

NIH3T3 cells were transfected with plasmids, pMTVHBx, pMTVAd12, pMTVE1A, pMTVE1B or pUC18 together with pRSVneo by the calcium phosphate method. Construction of the plasmid pMTVHBx will be described elsewhere. In pMTVHBx, the *HBx* gene is under the control of mouse mammary tumor virus (MMTV)-long terminal repeat (LTR), and its expression is regulated with dexamethasone (DEX) (Fig. 1). Cells were then

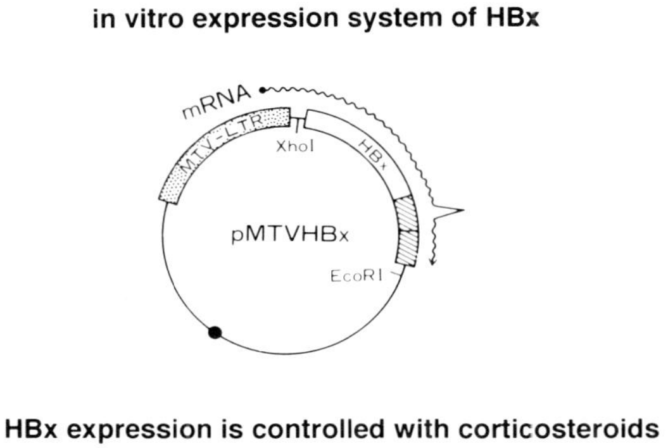

Fig. 1. Plasmid pMTVHBx which was introduced into NIH3T3 cells. *HBx* gene is under the control of mouse mammary tumor virus (MMTV)-long terminal repeat (LTR), and its expression is regulated with dexamethasone.

selected with geneticin (G418, GIBCO Laboratories, Grand Island, NY, USA), and selected clones were analyzed for introduced genes by the polymerase chain reaction (PCR) method or Southern blotting.

DNA, RNA and protein analysis

Southern, Northern or Western blotting was used as described previously [8].

Results

Non-neoplastic liver in HBx transgenic mice (Fig. 2)

We focused our analysis on male mice of the H9 lineage that had high levels of *HBx* gene expression [7]. Twenty-eight animals were examined, beginning at 4 weeks. At 4 weeks, the livers of the transgenic mice appeared normal. At 2 months, the mice began to show foci of altered hepatocytes, concentrated mainly in centrilobular areas in which foci consisted of relatively large hepatocytes with vacuolations poorly stained with hematoxylin-eosin staining in the cytoplasm. These vacuolations were periodic acid-Schiff staining positive and were considered to contain glycogen. These vacuolated cells expressed relatively higher levels of HBx protein than those around the portal vein areas. No elevation of serum alanine aminotransferase was observed at the age of 10 months.

High-level expression of HBx gene was already detected in the livers from 1-month-old mice in which the foci of vacuolated hepatocytes had not emerged. At 7 to 10 months, small clusters of dysplastic hepatocytes with large nuclei and increased chromatin appeared within the foci, but the foci did not expand and neoplastic changes were not observed until 12 months. Around 12 months large areas of dysplastic hepatocytes occasionally appeared, accompanied by small nodules that were presumably precursors of adenomas. Also found at this age was hyperplasia that demonstrated higher levels of *HBx* gene expression than the surrounding areas. Subsequently, adenomas and HCCs appeared, beginning at 13 months. Among 37 male mice of the H9 line that had died or were killed because of sickness, 31 (84%) were found to have hepatic neoplasia, and in some animals they formed large masses.

Increased DNA synthesis in non-neoplastic liver

The 4-, 7- and 10-month-old transgenic mice that were assigned as tumor-free were labeled with BrdU intraperitoneally and examined for DNA synthesis in nuclei. All the transgenic mice treated demonstrated uptake of BrdU into the nuclei of hepatocytes in the altered foci around the central veins, in which the *HBx* gene was overexpressed in relationship to surrounding tissues. Age- and sex-matched nontransgenic litter mates that were treated by exactly the same method did not show any uptake of BrdU into nuclei.

DNA content analysis

DNA ploidy during the course of liver carcinogenesis as a consequence of the *HBx* gene expression was examined using a flow cytometer. In the 2-month-old transgenic mouse, a diploid peak, together with tetraploid and octaploid peaks, was detected in the liver cell nuclei, which showed no difference from a nontransgenic littermate. In contrast, in 4- and 7-month-old HBx transgenic mouse livers, tetraploid and octaploid populations decreased and several small aneuploid peaks appeared between diploid and tetraploid peaks.

Isolation and analysis of NIH3T3 cells expressing HBx gene in response to dexamethasone

We analyzed 11 out of 41 clones which had the plasmid pMTVHBx (named MTX cell lines), together with the clones with control plasmids. Six cell lines showed marked induction of HBx gene expression after DEX stimulation, while the remaining 5 lines had only a slight increase in HBx gene expression. The expression of HBx protein began to increase as early as 3 h after the addition of DEX, reached its peak at 6 h, and returned to the basal level after 24 h.

To determine the effect of HBx gene expression on the induction of cellular DNA synthesis in MTX cells, 11 lines of MTX cells and control cell lines were cultivated in two sets of Lab-tek chambers and maintained in a medium containing 0.1% FCS for 48 h. One set of chambers was labeled with BrdU for 1 h after 24 h incubation with DEX at a concentration of 10^{-6} M. Labeled cells were then stained with anti-BrdU monoclonal antibody and processed for visualization. The percentage of labeled cells increased significantly after DEX induction of HBx gene in MTX cells, while no increase was observed in control neomycin-selected NIH3T3 cells. In six of the MTX cell lines which had high levels of HBx protein with DEX stimulation, the percentage of labeled nuclei in the untreated cultures was 2–12% and increased to 8–37% after DEX stimulation, while in the remaining five cell lines the percentage increased very slightly, which is consistent with the low basal level and only slight induction of HBx gene expression in these cell lines. In five control cell lines, NIH3T3/neo-series, no increase of labeled nuclei was observed after the addition of DEX. Among other control cell lines, cells with pMTVE1A plasmid demonstrated increased DNA synthesis as described previously [9], while cells with pMTVE1B plasmid showed no increase despite the induction of E1B gene expression with DEX.

The progression of the cell cycle in MTX cell lines after the addition of DEX was also monitored by flow cytometry. After 18 h of treatment, the number of MTX cell lines in the S phase markedly increased with a concomitant decrease of cells in the G_0/G_1 phase. After 24 h, most of the cells entered into the S and G_2/M phase, and the cell cycle progressed further toward 48 h. In contrast, the majority of control neo-line cells remained in the G_0/G_1 phase after the addition of DEX.

Morphologically, MTX cell lines did not show the phenotype of transformed cells. The saturation densities of MTX cell lines were slightly higher than the parental NIH3T3 cells but comparable to those of NIH3T3/neo-control cell lines. None of the MTX cells or control NIH3T3/neo-cells induced tumors when inoculated into nude mice in spite of daily administration of DEX.

Discussion

We investigated the HBx transgenic mice from birth to the end of their life span to elucidate the consequences of HBx gene expression in hepatocytes which eventually lead to the development of HCC. There was no obvious cell death or regeneration process preceding the development of neoplasia, indicating that the mechanism of carcinogenesis is distinct from that in other transgenic mice harboring the HBV gene [10], in which continued cell death and regeneration are assumed to lead to the development of HCC [11].

In our analysis, low levels of HBx expression were insufficient for initiating tumor formation in mouse liver. This may explain the absence of tumor formation in other transgenic mice reported previously into which genomic or subgenomic HBV fragments were introduced as transgenes [12–14]. In the transgenic mice carrying the HBx gene only, under a heterologous regulatory

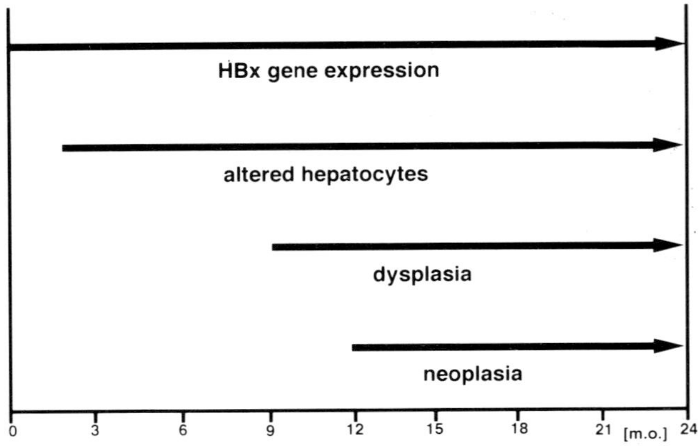

Fig. 2. Natural course of HBx transgenic mice. HBx gene expression starts from birth, and preneoplastic lesions appear from 2 months of age. Hepatocellular carcinoma finally develops from 13 months old. Horizontal axis indicates mouse age in months.

element [15], the expression of HBx gene was terminated by the age of 4 weeks, in contrast to the finding in our transgenic mice that HBx gene expression continued from 1 to at least 10 months of age, as shown by RNA blotting. Continued expression of more than a threshold level of HBx gene presumably at the appropriate sites in the liver, which were the areas around the central veins in our transgenic mice, may be necessary for development of HCC.

In the HBx transgenic mice, foci of hepatocytes with vacuolations in the cytoplasm appeared as early as age 2 months. These cells chiefly existed around the central veins, with the same subset of cells expressing relatively higher levels of HBx protein. An important finding is that these altered foci did not increase in size and no neoplastic change emerged until 10 months, although there appeared a small number of clusters of hepatocytes with large nuclei. Neoplasia finally appeared after 13 months (Fig. 2). Long incubation periods for tumor formation and the fact that only a small population of the altered foci developed into neoplasia indicate that at least one more genetic or epigenetic event is necessary for development of HCC in the HBx transgenic mice, which is also considered to be the case with other mice transgenic for oncogenes such as *myc* or *ras* [16].

Interestingly, some subsets of hepatocytes during this incubation period demonstrated increased DNA synthesis and aneuploid DNA contents. Increased DNA synthesis was observed in the cells around the central veins, which had relatively higher levels of HBx gene expression. It is not clear why HBx gene was expressed more highly in hepatocytes around the central veins, but it is noteworthy that there is a deviation of metabolism and enzyme distribution between hepatocytes around the portal and hepatic veins [17] and

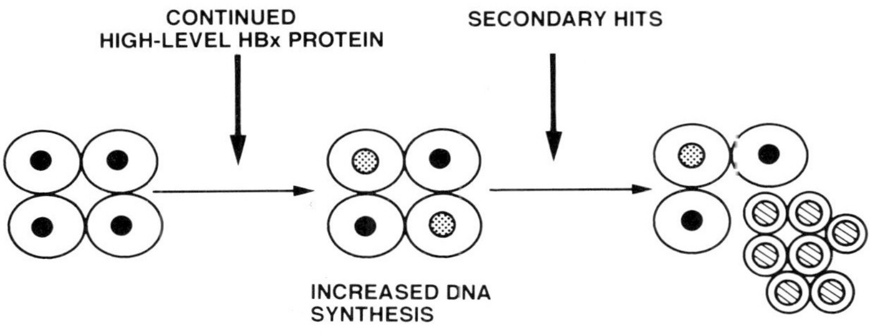

Fig. 3. The role of HBx gene in hepatocarcinogenesis in human hepatitis B virus infection (hypothesis).

that hepatocytes in the latter zone are not potentially proliferative [18]. The presence of aneuploid DNA contents suggests increased cell populations with DNA synthesis (S-phase) [19] or the existence of cells with chromosomal aberrations that are consistent with the livers of young transgenic mice being in the preneoplastic state as a result of HBx gene expression [20]. It is unclear why we could not see neoplastic changes in the liver for 8 months despite the existence of increased DNA synthesis in preneoplastic hepatocytes. It might be possible that coexisting apoptosis in preneoplastic foci accounts for this phenomenon, although we could not detect an increase of apoptotic bodies compared to normal control mice.

Our data with MTX cell lines clearly demonstrate that overexpression of HBx protein induces cell cycle progression in established culture cells. These HBx-expressing cells may be predisposed to transformation and may be subject to secondary hits which are independent from the events provoked by HBx protein. It is interesting to note that nuclear oncogenes such as the adenovirus early region 1a [9] or *c-myc* gene [21] have been known to possess mitogenic activity, which is the new property of HBx gene, and the mitogenic activity of these genes is considered to be closely related to their immortalized abilities [9]. In this sense, HBx gene might belong to nuclear-type oncogenes. Failure to transform NIH3T3 cells [22] and being a transcriptional transactivator are consistent with HBx gene being a potential nuclear-type oncogene. On the other hand, transgenic mouse studies have shown that growth factors such as TGFα are potential oncoproteins when their expression is deregulated in vivo [23]. In this context, the mitogenic activity itself of HBx protein, which was shown in the present study, may contribute to hepatocarcinogenesis in vivo. Alteration of cell growth cycle controls by HBx protein, resulting in continued cycling of cells under conditions which restrict the growth of normal cells, may be a major event in carcinogenesis in human HBV infection (Fig. 3).

Recently evidence has been accumulated which suggests the contribution of HBx protein to development of HCC in human HBV infection by means of immunostaining [24,25] or the RT-PCR method [26]. The relevance of HBx gene to hepatocarcinogenesis is now thus supported not only by the evidence in mice or culture cells but also by the data from human samples. Kekule et al. [22] have reported that HBx protein uses the PKC signaling pathway, which also mediates tumor promotion by growth factors, mitogens and phorbor esters. Vacuolated lesions in our mice, which – as mentioned earlier – resembled altered foci produced by carcinogens and showed increased DNA synthesis, might have been caused by HBx protein through the PKC pathway as by mitogens or tumor promoters [27]. In this context, HBx protein may function as a mitogen and make hepatocytes more susceptible to secondary events in hepatocarcinogenesis in human beings.

References

1. Beasley RP, Hwang L-Y. In: Vyas GN, Dienstag JL, Hoofnagle JH (eds) Viral Hepatitis and Liver Disease. Orlando: Grune and Stratton, 1984;209–224.
2. Tiollais P, Pourcell C, Dejean A. Nature 1985;317:489–495.
3. Tokino T, Fukushige T, Nakamura T et al. J Virol 1987;61:3848–3854.
4. Twu J-S, Schlomer R H. J Virol 1987;61:3448–3453.
5. Wollersheim M, Debelka U, Hofschneider PH. Oncogene 1988;3:545–552.
6. Kim C, Koike K, Saito I et al. Nature 1991;351:317–320.
7. Koike K, Moriya K, Iino S et al. Hepatology 1994;19:810–819.
8. Koike K, Hinrichs S, Isselbacher KJ et al. Proc Natl Acad Sci USA 1989;86:5615–5619.
9. Braithwaite AW, Cheetham BF, Li P et al. J Virol 1983;45:192–199.
10. Chisari FV, Klopchin KM, Moriyama T et al. Cell 1989;59:1145–1156.
11. Dunsford HA, Sell S, Chisari FV. Cancer Res 1990;50:3400–3407.
12. Araki K, Miyazaki J, Hino O et al. Proc Natl Acad Sci USA 1989;86:207–211.
13. Farza H, Hadchouel M, Scott J et al. J Virol 1988;62:4144–4152.
14. Burk RD, DeLoia JA, El Awady MK et al. J Virol 1988;62:649–654.
15. Lee TH, Finegold MJ, Shen RF et al. J Virol 1990;64:5939–5947.
16. Hanahan D. Ann Rev Genet 1988;22:479–519.
17. Scothorne RJ, MacSween RNM. Hepatology 1986;6:1050–1052.
18. Jungermann K, Katz N. Physiol Rev 1989;69:708–764.
19. Ornitz DM, Hammer RE, Messing A et al. Science 1978;238:188–193.
20. Reid BJ, Blount PL, Rubin CF et al. Gastroenterology 1992;102:1212–1219.
21. Armelin HA, Armelin MCS, Kelly K et al. Nature 1984;310:655–660.
22. Kekule AS, Lauer U, Weiss L et al. Nature 1993;361:742–745.
23. Lee GH, Merlino G, Fausto N. Cancer Res 1992;52:5162–5170.
24. Wang W, Lomdon WT, Feitelson MA. Cancer Res 1991;51:4971–4977.
25. Int J Cancer 1993;55:571–576.
26. Diamantis ID, McGandy CE, Chen T-J et al. J Hepatol 1992;15:400–403.
27. Nishizuka Y. Nature 1984;308:693–698.

Index of authors

Keyword index